Adjudicated Youth

Editor

LOUIS J. KRAUS

CHILD AND ADOLESCENT PSYCHIATRIC CLINICS OF NORTH AMERICA

www.childpsych.theclinics.com

Consulting Editor
HARSH K. TRIVEDI

January 2016 • Volume 25 • Number 1

ELSEVIER

1600 John F. Kennedy Boulevard • Suite 1800 • Philadelphia, Pennsylvania, 19103-2899

http://www.theclinics.com

CHILD AND ADOLESCENT PSYCHIATRIC CLINICS OF NORTH AMERICA Volume 25, Number 1
January 2016 ISSN 1056–4993, ISBN-13: 978-0-323-41443-2

Editor: Lauren Boyle
Developmental Editor: Kristen Helm

Child and Adolescent Psychiatric Clinics of North America (ISSN 1056-4993) is published quarterly by Elsevier Inc., 360 Park Avenue South, New York, NY 10010-1710. Months of issue are January, April, July, and October. Business and Editorial Offices: 1600 John F. Kennedy Boulevard, Suite 1800, Philadelphia, PA 19103-2899. Periodicals postage paid at New York, NY and additional mailing offices. Subscription prices are $310.00 per year (US individuals), $544.00 per year (US institutions), $100.00 per year (US students), $360.00 per year (Canadian individuals), $662.00 per year (Canadian institutions), $200.00 per year (Canadian students), $430.00 per year (international individuals), $662.00 per year (international institutions), and $200.00 per year (international students). International air speed delivery is included in all *Clinics* subscription prices. All prices are subject to change without notice. **POSTMASTER:** Send address changes to *Child and Adolescent Psychiatric Clinics of North America*, Elsevier Health Sciences Division, Subscription Customer Service, 3251 Riverport Lane, Maryland Heights, MO 63043. **Customer Service: 1-800-654-2452 (U.S. and Canada); 314-447-8871 (outside U.S. and Canada). Fax: 314-447-8029. E-mail:** JournalsCustomerService-usa@elsevier.com **(for print support) or** journalsonlinesupport-usa@elsevier.com **(for online support).**

Reprints. For copies of 100 or more of articles in this publication, please contact the Commercial Reprints Department, Elsevier Inc., 360 Park Avenue South, New York, New York 10010-1710 Tel.: 212-633-3874; Fax: 212-633-3820, E-mail: reprints@elsevier.com.

Child and Adolescent Psychiatric Clinics of North America is covered in *MEDLINE/PubMed (Index Medicus), ISI, SSCI, Research Alert, Social Search, Current Contents,* and *EMBASE/Excerpta Medica.*

Contributors

CONSULTING EDITOR

HARSH K. TRIVEDI, MD, MBA
Executive Director and Chief Medical Officer; Behavioral Health Vice Chair for Clinical Affairs; Associate Professor of Psychiatry, Vanderbilt University School of Medicine, Nashville, Tennessee

CONSULTING EDITOR EMERITUS

ANDRÉS MARTIN, MD, MPH

FOUNDING CONSULTING EDITOR

MELVIN LEWIS, MBBS, FRCPSYCH, DCH

EDITOR

LOUIS J. KRAUS, MD
Woman's Board Professor and Chief, Section of Child and Adolescent Psychiatry; Director, Autism Assessment, Research, Treatment and Services (AARTS) Center, Rush University Medical Center, Chicago, Illinois

AUTHORS

DALIA N. BALSAMO, MD
Clinical Fellow, Child Study Center, Yale School of Medicine, New Haven, Connecticut

ELIZABETH S. BARNERT, MD, MPH, MS
Department of Pediatrics, David Geffen School of Medicine, University of California Los Angeles, Los Angeles, California

ERAKA BATH, MD
Director, Child Forensic Services; Assistant Professor, Department of Psychiatry and Biobehavioral Sciences, Semel Institute for Neuroscience and Human Behavior, University of California Los Angeles, Los Angeles, California

MEKEILA COOK, PhD
Integrated Substance Abuse Programs, Department of Psychiatry and Biobehavioral Sciences, Semel Institute for Neuroscience and Human Behavior, University of California Los Angeles, Los Angeles, California

BRADLEY FREEMAN, MD
Assistant Professor of Clinical Psychiatry, Department of Psychiatry, Vanderbilt University School of Medicine, Nashville, Tennessee

SHUSHANIK GABOIAN, MSW
Associate Clinical Social Worker, Department of Neuroscience and Human Behavior, University of California Los Angeles, Los Angeles, California

ARTHA J. GILLIS, MD, PhD
Child and Adolescent Psychiatry Fellow, Department of Psychiatry and Biobehavioral Sciences, Semel Institute for Neuroscience and Human Behavior, University of California Los Angeles, Los Angeles, California

ROYA IJADI-MAGHSOODI, MD
Advanced Fellow in Women's Health, VA HSR&D Center for the Study of Healthcare Innovation, Implementation and Policy, VA Greater Los Angeles Healthcare System; Department of Medicine, David Geffen School of Medicine, University of California Los Angeles, Los Angeles, California

LOUIS J. KRAUS, MD
Woman's Board Professor and Chief, Section of Child and Adolescent Psychiatry; Director, Autism Assessment, Research, Treatment and Services (AARTS) Center, Rush University Medical Center, Chicago, Illinois

JACQUELINE LANDESS, MD, JD
Forensic Psychiatry Fellow, University of Colorado, Aurora, Colorado

SOO JUNG LEE, MD
Assistant Professor, Section of Child and Adolescent Psychiatry, Autism Assessment, Research, and Treatment Services (AARTS) Center, Rush University Medical Center, Chicago, Illinois

CAMILLA L. LYONS, MD, MPH
Clinical Assistant Professor, Department of Psychiatry, New York University School of Medicine, New York, New York

ANNE McBRIDE, MD
Assistant Clinical Professor of Psychiatry, Department of Psychiatry and Behavioral Sciences, University of California Davis Medical Center, Sacramento, California

BRITTANY PETERS, MD
Child and Adolescent Psychiatry Fellow, Department of Psychiatry, Vanderbilt University School of Medicine, Nashville, Tennessee

YANN B. PONCIN, MD
Assistant Professor, Child Study Center, Yale School of Medicine, New Haven, Connecticut

JOHN S. ROZEL, MD, MSL
Medical Director, Re:solve Crisis Network; Assistant Professor of Psychiatry, University of Pittsburgh School of Medicine; Adjunct Professor, University of Pittsburgh School of Law; Supervising Psychiatrist, Shuman Detention Center, Pittsburgh, Pennsylvania

EILEEN P. RYAN, DO
Associate Professor of Psychiatry and Neurobehavioral Sciences, Institute of Law, Psychiatry, and Public Policy, University of Virginia School of Medicine, Charlottesville, Virginia; Medical Director, Commonwealth Center for Children and Adolescents, Staunton, Virginia

SHAWN S. SIDHU, MD
Assistant Professor, Department of Psychiatry, University of New Mexico, Albuquerque, New Mexico

MATTHEW SOULIER, MD
Associate Clinical Professor of Psychiatry, Division of the Psychiatry and Law, University of California Davis Medical Center, Sacramento, California

SOFIA T. STEPANYAN, BA
Graduate Student, Developmental Psychology, Department of Psychology, University of California Riverside, Riverside, California

KEVIN WHITLEY, MD, MA
Southwood Psychiatric Hospital, Pittsburgh, Pennsylvania

SHAWN S. SIDHU, MD
Assistant Professor, Department of Psychiatry, University of New Mexico, Albuquerque, New Mexico

MATTHEW SOULIER, MD
Associate Clinical Professor of Psychiatry, Division of the Psychiatry and Law, University of California Davis Medical Center, Sacramento, California

SOFIA T. STEPANYAN, BA
Graduate Student, Developmental Psychology, Department of Psychology, University of California Riverside, Riverside, California

KEVIN WHITLEY, MD, MA
Southwood Psychiatric Hospital, Pittsburgh, Pennsylvania

Contents

of much discussion. With serious crimes, juvenile delinquents may be transferred from juvenile court to adult criminal court; this practice became more prevalent in the past century. However, growing knowledge of adolescent development has mitigated the culpability of youth offenders and resulted in judicial decisions influential to juvenile dispositions.

Juvenile Competency to Stand Trial 49

Sofia T. Stepanyan, Shawn S. Sidhu, and Eraka Bath

Competency to stand trial is interpreted as a protected due process right for all defendants and is defined as a defendant's fundamental knowledge and understanding of the criminal charges being filed, roles and procedures within the courtroom, and a general ability to work with the defense counsel. Questions of competency are most often raised by the judge, defense, or the prosecution, and competency evaluations are most often completed by psychiatrists or psychologists with forensic training or work experience. Mental illness, intellectual disability, developmental disorders, and developmental immaturity are the 4 main factors considered in most juvenile competency evaluations.

The Role of the Child and Adolescent Psychiatrist in the Adjudicatory Assessment 61

Camilla L. Lyons

When courts look to mental health professionals to help inform legal decisions, psychiatrists are key members of the skilled clinicians qualified to respond. Child and adolescent psychiatrists are in a unique position to apply their diagnostic acumen and expertise in psychopharmacology to adjudicatory assessments. Key components of these evaluations include diagnostic assessment, risk assessment, treatment amenability, and specific recommendations for available treatment. This article culls guidelines for adjudicatory assessments from the existing peer-reviewed literature, including the use of structured professional judgment tools, the avoidance of dual agency, and the measured use of juvenile psychopathy assessment tools.

Mental Health Care of Detained Youth and Solitary Confinement and Restraint Within Juvenile Detention Facilities 71

Kevin Whitley and John S. Rozel

Justice-involved youth are a complex and heterogeneous population with extremely high rates of mental disorder, trauma, and numerous other psychosocial stressors. Although working with this population has several challenges it can be highly rewarding for clinicians and a powerful opportunity for prevention of subsequent problems. Psychosocial interventions remain some of the most robust and effective interventions targeting specific developmental deficits common in this population. Medication treatment is also often appropriate. Seclusion may be clinically appropriate in some cases and is seen as distinct from disciplinary interventions such as isolation or solitary confinement, which are generally not appropriate.

Juvenile Sex Offenders **81**

Eileen P. Ryan

Public policy has tended to treat juvenile sex offenders (JSOs) as adult sex offenders in waiting, despite research that contradicts this notion. Although as a group, JSOs are more similar to general delinquents than to adult sex offenders, atypical sexual interests and sexual victimization during childhood may be a pathway for sexual offending that differentiates some JSOs from their nonsexually delinquent peers. Developmental considerations must be considered in risk assessment evaluations of these youth. This article reviews theories of sexual offending in youth, risk factors for juvenile offending and reoffending, psychopathology in JSOs, risk assessment, and treatment.

Juvenile Firesetting **99**

Brittany Peters and Bradley Freeman

Juvenile firesetting is a significant cause of morbidity and mortality in the United States. Male gender, substance use, history of maltreatment, interest in fire, and psychiatric illness are commonly reported risk factors. Interventions that have been shown to be effective in juveniles who set fires include cognitive behavior therapy and educational interventions, whereas satiation has not been shown to be an effective intervention. Forensic assessments can assist the legal community in adjudicating youth with effective interventions. Future studies should focus on consistent assessment and outcome measures to create more evidence for directing evaluation and treatment of juvenile firesetters.

Understanding and Responding to the Needs of Commercially Sexually Exploited Youth: Recommendations for the Mental Health Provider **107**

Roya Ijadi-Maghsoodi, Mekeila Cook, Elizabeth S. Barnert, Shushanik Gaboian, and Eraka Bath

Mental health providers are frequently at the forefront of addressing the multifaceted needs of commercially sexually exploited youth. This article provides an overview of the definition of commercial sexual exploitation of children and relevant legislation including the shift toward decriminalization of commercially sexually exploited youth. To provide clinicians with tools needed to deliver competent care to this population, a review of risk factors for commercial sexual exploitation of children and the role of the clinician in identification, assessment, and treatment of commercially sexually exploited youth are discussed.

Community-Based Alternatives to Incarceration and Assessment and Community-Based Planning for Probation/Community-Based Alternative **123**

Dalia N. Balsamo and Yann B. Poncin

There is growing concern regarding the current treatment of juvenile offenders within the justice system. Most mental health professionals would agree that it is best to adopt a rehabilitative approach toward delinquent youths, but current practices do not always follow this principle. Youth

incarceration is a costly and often debilitative process. There is growing evidence for community-based alternatives that aim to rehabilitate juvenile delinquents. Some of these interventions have proved to be successful in the prevention of delinquent acts.

Index **129**

CHILD AND ADOLESCENT PSYCHIATRIC CLINICS

FORTHCOMING ISSUES

April 2016
Prevention of Mental Health Disorders: Principles and Implementation
Aradhana Bela Sood and James Hudziak, *Editors*

July 2016
Substance Use Disorders, Part I
Ray Hsiao and Leslie Walker, *Editors*

October 2016
Substance Use Disorders, Part II
Ray Hsiao and Paula Riggs, *Editors*

RECENT ISSUES

October 2015
Global Mental Health
Paramjit T. Joshi and Lisa M. Cullins, *Editors*

July 2015
Family-Based Treatment in Child and Adolescent Psychiatry
Michelle L. Rickerby and Thomas A. Roesler, *Editors*

April 2015
School Mental Health
Margaret M. Benningfield and Sharon Hoover Stephan, *Editors*

Preface
Juvenile Delinquency

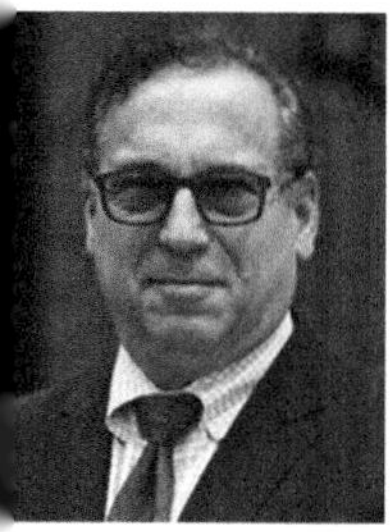

Louis J. Kraus, MD
Editor

This issue of *Child and Adolescent Psychiatric Clinics of North America* focuses on juvenile delinquency, advancements over the past century, current proceedings, and ongoing dilemmas. With the recognition of children, their vulnerability, and unique needs delineating them from adults, many policies and services have been established to protect and meet the needs of children. These changes also encompassed youth delinquency. The first youth detention center, The New York House of Refuge, was developed and the first juvenile court was established in Chicago during the nineteenth century. In the following century, growing interest in the specific needs of juveniles has helped the juvenile justice system better cater to this population.

Juvenile court has always centered on a balance between the police power, protecting the constituents of one's state, and a *Parens Patriae* model. Unlike adult court, the juvenile courts emphasized rehabilitation and not punishment with the expectation that, if appropriate interventions are available, rehabilitation can occur. Juvenile courts remain a civil, not a criminal, system. Juveniles are adjudicated, not tried; they are found delinquent, not guilty, and they are placed, not incarcerated.

Youths in the juvenile system compared with the general population have higher special education and mental health needs and are some of the most vulnerable children in our country. Educational accommodations and mental health care are inadequately provided in the community, which may increase the likelihood of recidivism. However, with appropriate interventions, the majority of youths in the juvenile system may be helped.

The pendulum has swung back and forth from meeting the needs of delinquent youth to punishment. This ongoing debate and reconsiderations for a punitive model demand the much needed advocacy in juvenile justice. As a society, this vulnerable population has been largely ignored. This issue of *Child and Adolescent Psychiatric Clinics of North America* allows us to refocus on this group in need.

Topics focus on demographics. There has been a plateau for significant delinquent behavior. At the same time, there continues to be concern over minority overrepresentation within the juvenile justice system. Understanding the civil and constitutional

Child Adolesc Psychiatric Clin N Am 25 (2016) xiii–xiv
http://dx.doi.org/10.1016/j.chc.2015.09.001

rights of adjudicated youth continues to be at the forefront of local, state, and federal cases.

A number of articles focus on the mental health screening and related issues of culpability of juveniles within juvenile court, including transfer/ waiver cases, juvenile competency to stand trial, and the role of the child and adolescent psychiatrist in the adjudicatory assessment. We know that upwards of 60% to 70% of detained youth have a significant mental health diagnosis, yet only a small percentage of them gets adequate treatment. The mental health care of detained youth is extremely important because of the high percentage of youth with mental health concerns. An article on the deleterious effects and impact of solitary confinement and restraint within juvenile detention facilities and the resultant changes that are occurring is quite timely. Further articles within the issue focus on more specific areas of juvenile offenses, including juvenile sex offenders, juvenile firesetting, and sexually exploited youth. There is a focus on community-based alternatives to incarceration, assessment, and community-based planning for probation.

The important topics covered by various articles in this issue help us to understand the complexity of the juvenile justice system and its continual need for a thoughtful process integrating social, political, and research aspects into its practice. It is of great importance that these youth are protected with their civil and constitutional rights while having accessible medical and mental health services. I would like to thank all of the authors for their wonderful articles, and I hope that you find this issue informative.

Louis J. Kraus, MD
Child and Adolescent Psychiatry
Rush University Medical Center
1645 West Jackson Street, Suite 603
Chicago, IL 60612, USA

E-mail address:
louis_kraus@rush.edu

Demographics

Artha J. Gillis, MD, PhD[a,*], Eraka Bath, MD[b]

KEYWORDS

- Disproportionate minority contact • Disproportionate minority confinement
- Juvenile delinquency • Racial disparities

KEY POINTS

- Disproportionate minority contact (DMC) has persisted over the past 20 to 30 years despite legislation intended to reduce this problem.
- Several individual, family, community, institutional, and sociolegal factors explain the presence and persistence of DMC.
- To reduce DMC, intervention strategies must address factors in multiple domains.
- Although DMC remains a problem on a national level, several jurisdictions have instituted interventions that successfully reduced DMC.
- More research is needed on the causes of DMC in multiple ethnic groups over the life course in order to inform the development of more broadly effective interventions.

INTRODUCTION

In 2013, juvenile courts nationwide processed 1,058,500 cases. Of the youth processed in juvenile court, 76% were male and 24% were female. Sixty-two percent were white, 35% were black, and less than 3% were American Indian or Asian/Native Hawaiian/Pacific Islander. Most were between the ages of 15 and 17 years (**Fig. 1**).[1]

Definition

Disproportionate minority contact (DMC) occurs when the proportion of African American, Hispanic, southeast Asian, Pacific Islander, Native American, and other disadvantaged ethnic minority youth at any given stage in the juvenile justice process exceeds the proportion of their respective group in the general population and exceeds white youth at the same stage in the juvenile justice process.[2–4] In

Disclosures: Dr A.J. Gillis has nothing to disclose. Dr E. Bath receives funding from the NIMH (2P20 MD000182) and the Los Angeles County Department of Probation.
[a] Department of Psychiatry and Biobehavioral Sciences, Semel Institute for Neuroscience and Human Behavior, University of California Los Angeles, 760 Westwood Plaza, Room C8-193, Los Angeles, CA 90024, USA; [b] Child Forensic Services, Department of Psychiatry and Biobehavioral Sciences, UCLA Neuropsychiatric Institute, University of California Los Angeles, 300 Medical Plaza, Room 1243, Los Angeles, CA 90095, USA
* Corresponding author.
E-mail address: agillis@mednet.ucla.edu

Child Adolesc Psychiatric Clin N Am 25 (2016) 1–17
http://dx.doi.org/10.1016/j.chc.2015.08.001 childpsych.theclinics.com
1056-4993/16/$ – see front matter

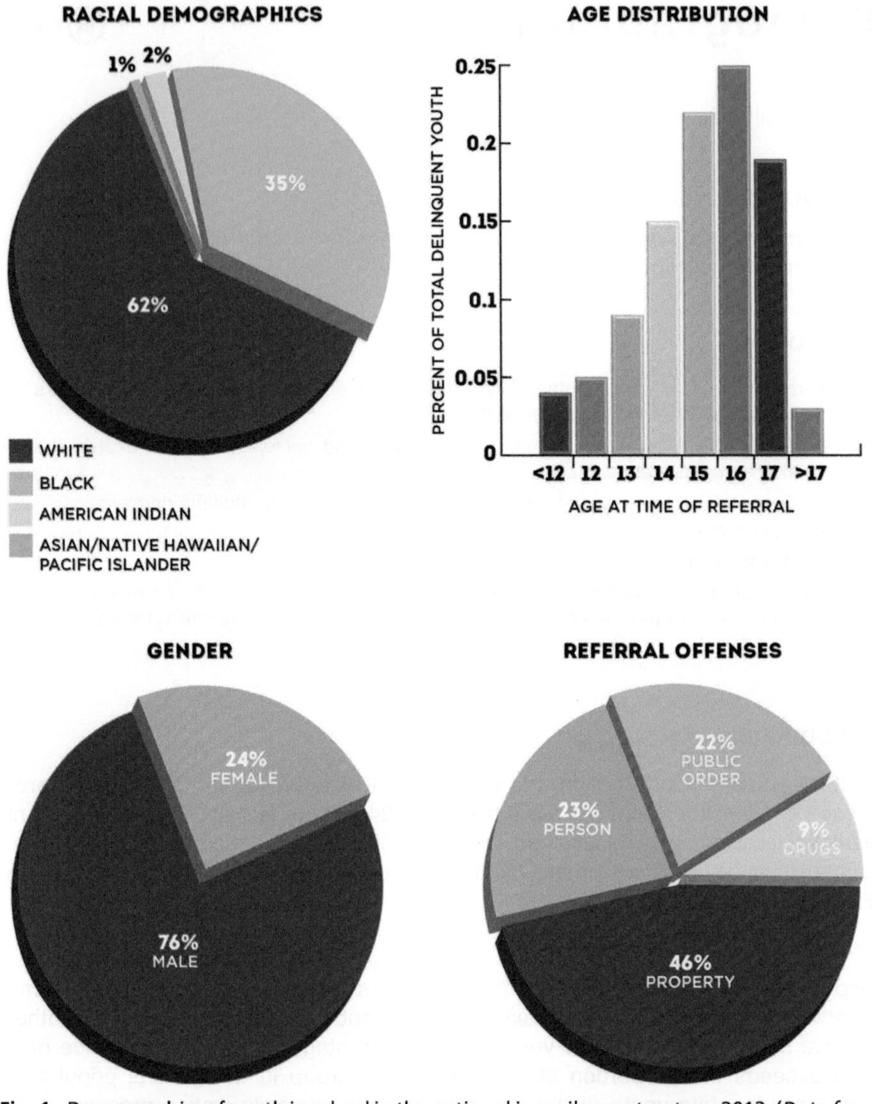

Fig. 1. Demographics of youth involved in the national juvenile court system, 2013. (*Data from* The Office of Juvenile Justice and Delinquency Prevention. Available at: http://www.ojjdp.gov/ojstatbb/. Accessed June 10, 2015.)

2013, 3 times as many black youth between the ages of 10 and 17 years were in the juvenile justice system, relative to their proportion in the general population, compared with white youth.[1] Hispanic, southeast Asian, Pacific Islander, and Native American youth are over-represented in some stages of the juvenile justice system, as well.[4–6] Several studies relate DMC to several individual, social, and system factors; its presence suggests racial disparities in society. It also suggests disparities in the treatment of minority youth in the juvenile justice system compared with white youth with similar individual and social risk factors, including risk factors for involvement in crime.[2]

Historical Legislative Trends and Shifts in the Juvenile Justice System

In order to understand the origins of DMC, it is helpful to examine the historical shifts in legislation and philosophies toward juvenile delinquency and juvenile court proceedings. In the 1960s and 1970s, the United States Supreme Court ruled in several cases involving juvenile delinquency proceedings and expanded civil rights for youth in the juvenile justice system. For example, in *Kent v United States* (1966), the Court formalized the process by which a juvenile defendant could be waived to adult criminal court and required juvenile courts to provide more due process when making such decisions.[7] In the case of *In re Gault* (1967), the Court granted many of the same due process protections found in criminal court to juvenile delinquency proceedings, including the right to confront witnesses, the right against self-incrimination, and the right to appropriate notification of the charges.[8] However, despite substantial gains in due process protections, the Just Deserts sentencing movement, which focused on offender accountability and punishment, emerged in the 1970s. As a result, juvenile courts began to shift their focus from rehabilitation to retribution.[9,10]

In many ways, Congress may have sought to shift the pendulum from retribution back to rehabilitation with a developmentally informed orientation toward juvenile culpability when it passed the Juvenile Justice and Delinquency Prevention (JJDP) Act in 1974.[11,12] The primary goals of the JJDP Act of 1974 were to deinstitutionalize status offenses and to remove juveniles from adult correctional facilities.[6] This law also created the Office of Juvenile Justice and Delinquency Prevention.

However, in the mid-1980s through the early 1990s, rates of serious juvenile crime increased. The Juvenile Violent Crime Index increased throughout this period and peaked in 1994.[13] Expectedly, juvenile justice courts across the nation processed an increasing number of delinquency cases.[13]

The public attributed the increase in crime in the 1980s to the urbanization of African Americans, and politicians fanned public panic by promising to crack down on increases in youth crime with laws that would get tough on crime.[5,9] Legislators responded to this shift in public opinion by proposing and passing laws outlining new policies relating to the possession, manufacture, and sale of crack cocaine. Because the use and sale of crack cocaine was more prevalent in African American communities, such laws disproportionately affected minority, and specifically African American, communities.[5]

In 1988, the Coalition of Juvenile Justice raised awareness of DMC in the juvenile justice system in its annual report to Congress, entitled *A Delicate Balance*.[12,14] When Congress amended the JJDP Act in 1988, they focused on "reducing and eliminating the over-representation of minority youth in detention and corrections facilities" and required states to address disproportionate minority confinement in their plans as a condition of funding.[12] In 1992, Congress amended the JJDP Act again, raising the focus on DMC to 1 of 4 core requirements for grant-funding eligibility.[12]

Between the early 1990s and the mid-2000s, the rates of juvenile crime continued to increase. Between 1990 and 1997, the rate of juvenile arrests for drug abuse violations increased by 145%.[13] By 2004, the number of youth detained in facilities awaiting court proceedings increased by 47%, compared with the number of youth detained in 1985. Over this same time period, the number of formal charges filed by district attorneys in the juvenile justice system increased from 45% to 57%, and the number of cases adjudicated or waived to criminal court increased from 29% of referred cases to 38% of these cases. The rates of formal probation and residential placement increased as well.[13]

In 1994, Congress passed the Safe and Drug-Free Schools and Communities Act (SDFSCA), which mandated severe punishment for disruptive students. The Gun-Free Schools Act, a subpart of the SDFSCA, mandated a minimum 1-year school expulsion by school districts of any student found in possession of a gun. Soon, zero tolerance policies proliferated and school districts began to mandate expulsion for hate speech, harassment, fighting in school, and dress code violations.[15] Subsequent studies showed that minority youth were more likely to be suspended for disruptive, nonviolent behavior,[16] and that African American and Latino students bear the brunt of zero tolerance policies.[17]

When Congress amended the JJDP Act in 2002, it broadened DMC from disproportionate minority confinement to disproportionate minority contact and required that states examine possible disproportionate representation of minority youth at 9 decision points in the juvenile justice process (**Fig. 2**). They also required intervention strategies that address system improvements in addition to prevention of juvenile delinquency (**Table 1**).

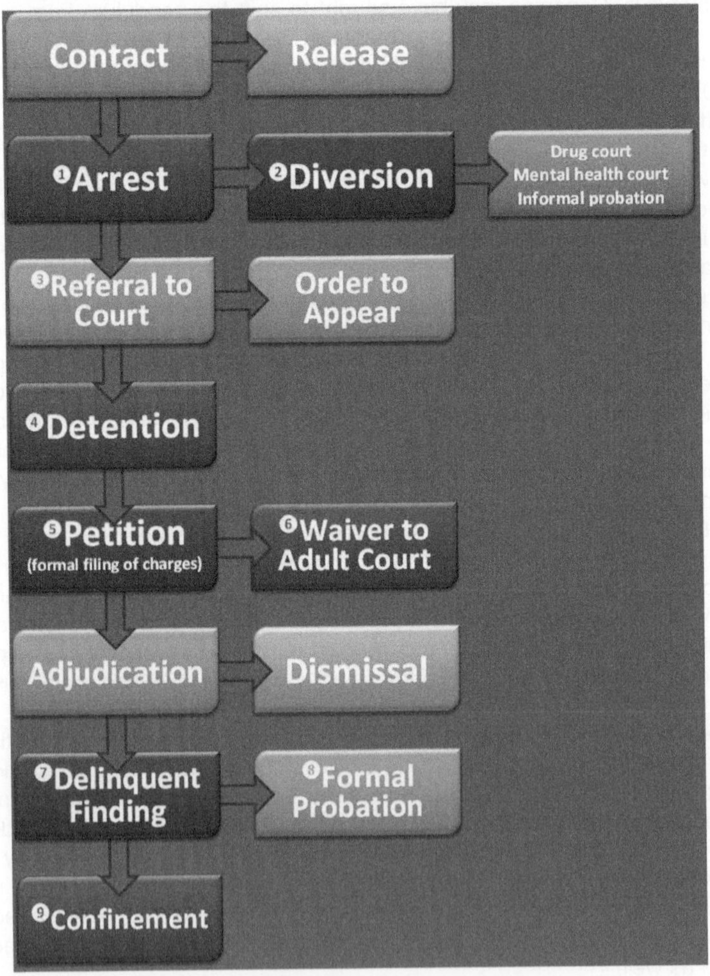

Fig. 2. Stages in the juvenile justice process.

Table 1
Key rulings and legislation related to DMC

Year	Ruling/Law	Significance
1966	*Kent v United States*	Formalized the process of waiver to criminal court
1967	*In re Gault*	Extended due process protections to juvenile delinquency proceedings
1974	JJDP Act	Deinstitutionalized status offenses; removed juveniles from adult correctional facilities
1988	First amendment of the JJDP Act	Required states to address DMC as a condition of funding
1992	Second amendment of the JJDP Act	Raised focus on DMC to a core requirement for grant funding
1994	SDFSCA	Mandated severe punishment for disruptive students
1994	Gun-Free Schools Act (subpart of SDFSCA)	Mandated a minimum 1-year school expulsion by school districts of any student found in possession of a gun
2002	Third amendment of the JJDP Act	Broadened focus of DMC from disproportionate minority confinement to disproportionate minority contact

THEORIES EXPLAINING DISPROPORTIONATE MINORITY CONTACT

Differential Involvement in Crime

One prominent theory suggests that the disproportionate involvement in criminal activity by minority youth, relative to white youth, explains the disproportionate representation of minority youth in the juvenile justice system.[5] Proponents of this theory suggest that minority youth commit more serious crimes, which are more likely to be reported, increasing the likelihood of being arrested. The difference in arrest rates explains the differences in rates of juvenile justice processing, including the difference in rates of postadjudication confinement.

Official police records and self-report surveys suggest that African American and Hispanic youth may be more involved in serious violent crimes than white youth.[5] One study found that African American youth were one-third more likely than white youth to commit a violent crime by the age of 17 years.[15]

However, in many studies, black and white youth reported similar amounts of illicit drug use.[5] In the National Household Survey on Drug Abuse, white youth (aged 12–17 years) reported selling drugs one-third more frequently than black youth.[18,19] In a study examining the risks and needs of status offenders in a large, Midwestern, metropolitan county, African American status offenders were "vastly"[20] over-represented in the juvenile justice system, although white status offenders displayed significantly greater risk across a variety of domains, including legal risks, educational risks, and risks of mental illness and substance abuse (**Fig. 3**).[20]

Therefore, differences in involvement in crime do not completely explain DMC in the juvenile justice system, especially given that the literature documents several areas in which white youth have greater risk of involvement that may potentiate legal contact. In a meta-analysis by Pope and Feyerherm,[22] racial differences in juvenile justice processing could not be explained solely by the legal characteristics of the youth. Approximately two-thirds of the studies reviewed in the meta-analysis indicated that racial status played a role at various stages of the juvenile justice process.[21,22] Further, studies show that zero tolerance policies in schools contribute to the school-to-prison pipeline.[15,23] The perception of minority youth as being more problematic and disruptive resulted in differential administration of punishments and sanctions, including

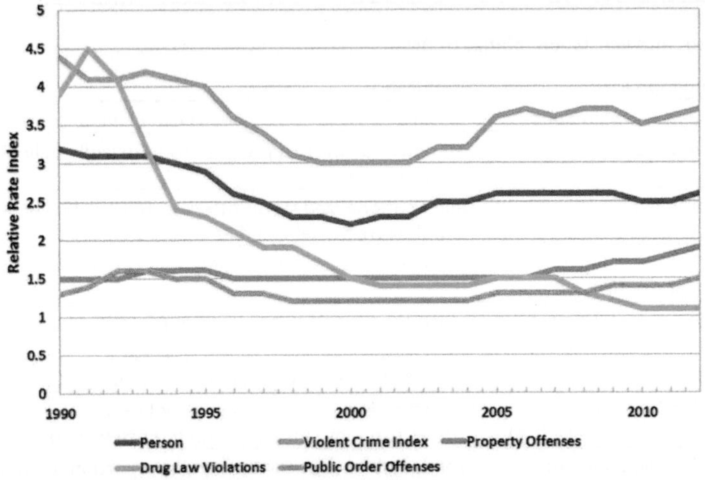

Fig. 3. Trends in the national relative rate index between 1990 to 2013 by category of crime. (*Data from* The Office of Juvenile Justice and Delinquency Prevention. Available at: http://www.ojjdp.gov/ojstatbb/. Accessed June 12, 2015.)

suspensions and expulsions. Since the institution of zero tolerance policies, the rates of school suspension and expulsions increased disproportionately for minority youth and in schools with higher minority youth populations.[15,24] Youth who are suspended or expelled are vulnerable, are often left unsupervised, and fall behind on schoolwork, increasing their risk of dropping out and potentiating their risk for delinquency.[23,25,26] As one study concluded, "there simply isn't any support for the notion that, given the same set of circumstances, African American kids act out to a greater degree than other kids."[15]

Differential Selection and Processing in the Juvenile Justice System

African American, Hispanic/Latino, Native American, southeast Asian American, and Pacific Islander youth are represented disproportionately at every stage of the juvenile justice system.[4–6] Even when referred for the same offense, African American youth are more likely than white youth to be formally charged, sentenced to residential facilities, and waived to adult criminal court.[5] In schools, African American students are more likely than white students to be suspended, expelled, or arrested for the same kind of conduct. Further, African American students receive harsher discipline for less serious offenses, such as disrespect, excessive noise, threats, and loitering.[15]

In a study examining factors that influence decision making in the juvenile justice system, individual offender characteristics, family and school contexts, and legal variables independently had a significant impact on decision making at intake. However, after the other variables were held constant, a main effect of race remained.[3] Race also affected assessments of family structure in this study: African American youth from single-parent homes were at a disadvantage at intake relative to white youth from single-parent homes.[3] In another study, black youth were more likely than white youth[6] to be detained pending referral to court, related to decisions made during bail hearings.[5] In a review of studies of youth charged with felonies in criminal courts in 40 of the largest jurisdictions in the country, black youth were more likely than white youth to be waived to adult criminal court. Although the overall percentage of waivers from juvenile court to adult criminal court remained constant at 1.4% between 1985 and 1995, the percentage of white youth waived to criminal court decreased from 57% to 51%, whereas the percentage of African American youth waived to criminal court increased from 41% to 46%.[6] In general, most youth waived to criminal court did not have serious violent charges. Instead, they were charged with offenses that are typically handled in juvenile court, suggesting differential treatment. For example, black youth with drug charges were waived at 5 times the rate of white youth with similar charges despite substantially higher self-reports of drug behavior by white youth relative to black youth.[18] More than 40% of the black youth waived to adult criminal court for felony offenses were not convicted, suggesting that the cases in general, and the case for waiver to adult criminal court more specifically, were not evidentially strong.[18]

Differences in policing

The juvenile justice system affords law enforcement wide discretion. Knowledge of a youth's prior record in addition to a youth's racial appearance, grooming and "demeanor that officers associated with 'true' delinquent boys" likely influences this discretion.[5] Perceptions by law enforcement personnel may influence their estimation of risks of reoffense by youth and, therefore, recommendations about detention and sentencing.

Because of get-tough laws and antigang policies, law enforcement may target certain crimes and certain communities.[2,5] These practices may affect minority youth or communities disproportionately, effectively increasing their contact with the juvenile justice system.[5]

Zero tolerance policies have also led to increased surveillance and policelike presence in many urban schools, increasing the places and situations in which youth have contact with law enforcement.[23] Schools with on-site law enforcement increase the risk of unnecessary involvement of their students with the juvenile justice system, because behaviors that were previously resolved by school administrators become criminalized. Further, law enforcement officers frequently lack expertise in development, education, or mental health. However, they make decisions on matters that were previously under the purview of trained educational administrators.[27] Youth who are suspended or expelled are vulnerable and are often left unsupervised, fall behind on their schoolwork, and therefore are more likely to drop out, further potentiating their risk for delinquency.[25]

Judicial discretion

Historically, the juvenile justice system served as a rehabilitative mechanism for youth offenders. With the focus on get-tough legislation beginning in the 1980s, it became more retributive and now serves dual goals.[4,9] As such, judges and other juvenile justice personnel practice with great discretion, often selecting between retribution and rehabilitation in individual cases. In addition, different juvenile justice personnel may be more or less concerned with retribution versus rehabilitation. The discretion that various juvenile justice personnel exercise may lead to disproportionate treatment of minority youth offenders relative to white youth offenders. For example, as cited in a report by Building Blocks for Youth, most studies in a meta-analysis examining race and the juvenile justice system concluded that race affects decisions negatively at multiple stages in the juvenile justice process.[28] Specifically, in a study examining more than 2500 cases involving white, African American, and Latino youth in 18 jurisdictions over a 6-month period, 43% of African American youth and 37% of Latino youth were sentenced to incarceration, compared with 26% of white youth, even when controlling for offense type.[29] Similarly, the National Council on Crime and Delinquency reported that African American youth were 6 times more likely and Latino youth were 3 times more likely to be incarcerated than white youth with similar backgrounds and charges.[28]

Prosecutors tend to value retribution more than rehabilitation. They place high priority on convictions and public safety.[3] They base their decisions about charges largely on evidentiary strength and crime severity. One study found that race is not typically a direct consideration in selection of charges. However, race does interact with crime severity: African American youth accused of felony offenses are more likely than similarly situated white youth to be formally charged.[3]

Further, prosecutors may waive youth offenders to adult criminal court through statutory exclusion or through prosecutorial discretion. Although prosecutors have expertise in selecting charges, some of which require mandatory waivers to adult criminal court, and in evaluating the evidentiary strength of a case, they do not own expertise in deciding whether to try a youth as a juvenile or as an adult.[9] However, in a review of data on youth waived to adult criminal court in 40 of the largest jurisdictions in the country, 80% of black youth were waived through statutory exclusion or by prosecutorial waiver, bypassing the need for a judicial hearing. Typically, forensically trained mental health professions inform such decisions, based on evaluations of amenability to rehabilitation and other considerations.[18,30]

During sentencing decisions, judges often consider an offender's amenability to treatment without the benefit of a standardized or objective assessment. Because of their subjectivity, these decisions may not be accurate, consistent, or uniform.[9] For example, in a study examining factors influencing decision making in the juvenile justice system, researchers found that only legal variables, such as the type of charge and the severity of the crime, influenced decisions about adjudication, except if the youth offender was African American. In these cases, the offender's prior record also influenced the adjudicatory decision.[3]

Cumulative effects of differential decision making in the juvenile justice system

Decisions at each stage of the juvenile justice process are not exclusive of previous or subsequent decisions, from arrest to disposition. The effects of differential decision making can accumulate. For example, in 1997 to 1998, black youth represented 15% of the general youth population, but 26% of the youth arrested, 31% of the youth referred for formal charges, 44% of the youth detained pending the hearing of their cases, 46% of the youth waived to adult criminal court, and 58% of youth sentenced to serve time in state prison.[21] In 2013, black youth still represented 15% of the general youth population, 30% of the youth arrested, 31% of the youth referred for formal charges, 42% of the youth detained pending hearing, and 58% of the youth waived to adult criminal court (**Figs. 4** and **5**).

Combined Effects of Differential Involvement in Crime and Differential Selection and Processing in the Juvenile Justice System

Neither differential involvement in crime nor differential selection and processing in the juvenile justice system fully explain the presence and persistence of DMC. Further, it is difficult to determine the relative weight of either theory in explaining the presence of disparities in the juvenile justice system, and neither theory is exclusive of the other. Differential involvement may influence differential selection and processing. The debate between these two theories remains at a "conceptual and methodological impasse."[5]

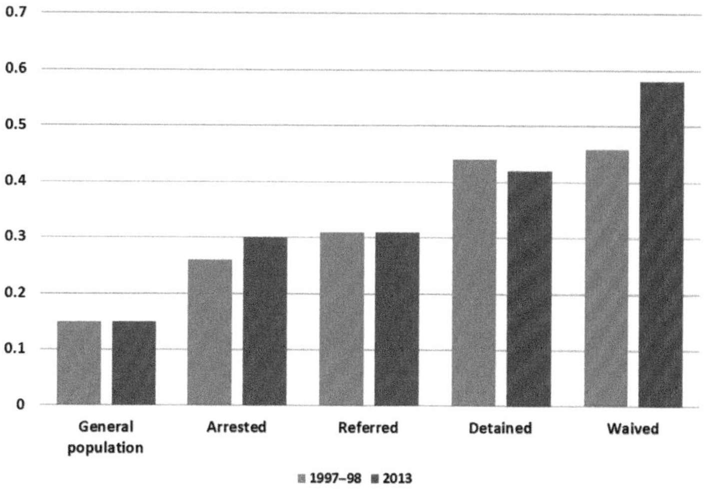

Fig. 4. Representation of African American youth in the juvenile justice system, 1997 to 98 and 2013. (*Data from* Kakar S. Understanding the causes of disproportionate minority contact: results of focus group discussions. J Crim Justice 2006;34:369–81; and The DMC Databook. Available at: http://www.ojjdp.gov/ojstatbb/dmcdb/. Accessed June 12, 2015.)

Psychosocial factors

Many studies attribute juvenile crime, in general, to family, social, community, educational, and other individual risk factors,[21] such as poor access to health care or untreated mental illness, which neither theory takes into account.

Individual factors

Between 65% and 75% of youth entering the juvenile justice system experience mental health disorders,[31,32] a rate that is 2 to 3 times higher than that of youth in

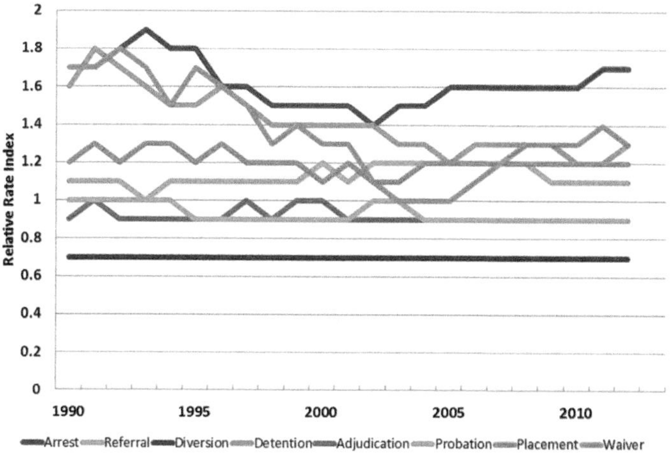

Fig. 5. Trends in the national relative rate index between 1990 to 2012, by stage in the juvenile justice process. (*Data from* The Office of Juvenile Justice and Delinquency Prevention. Available at: http://www.ojjdp.gov/ojstatbb/. Accessed June 12, 2015.)

the community.[25] The prevalence of psychiatric disorders for youth processed in the adult criminal court is even higher than the prevalence of psychiatric disorders for youth processed in the juvenile court.[33]

Multiple studies have compared differences in rates of mental health and substance abuse problems in different ethnic groups. White youth report the highest rates of psychiatric disorders in general, and substance abuse disorders more specifically. Although African American youth report the lowest rates of psychiatric and substance abuse disorders, both during and after detention,[25,34–36] their rate of psychiatric disorders remains high. Further, male African American youth experience more environmental stressors than male white youth.[24]

Poor access to health care is common for youth entering the juvenile justice system.[25] Substantiated reports of childhood maltreatment, a history of mental health problems, and a history of a learning disorder are risk factors for later juvenile justice involvement.[25,31] On entering the juvenile justice system, the presence of psychiatric disorders may be factored into decisions regarding disposition.[25]

Race may be indirectly associated with access to mental health care for youth involved in the juvenile justice system.[31] Although rates of psychiatric disorders may be lower in minority youth involved in the juvenile justice system, minority and low-income youth experience more barriers to mental health care,[31] making their access to mental health care even poorer than that of other youth in the juvenile justice system.[25,31,37] In addition, their symptoms may be less detected,[38] which may partially explain why minority youth have lower odds of accessing mental health care after detention, compared with white youth.[25,31,33] Further, African American youth experience learning disorders at a higher rate. Therefore, African American youth with learning disorders likely experience barriers to treatment at a greater rate than they would based on race or educational impairment alone.

Minority youth with psychiatric disorders are more likely than white youth to be placed in the juvenile justice system than they are to be diverted to the community for treatment.[31,37] To complicate access to mental health care further, the environment of out-of-home placements may exacerbate psychiatric disorders.[31] Although there is limited treatment in the community, mental health care resources in the juvenile justice system are often limited in breadth and scope.[25] Further, youth in the juvenile justice system often experience multiple psychiatric comorbidities.[33] Therefore, poor access to mental health care is likely a critical factor in the relative increase in morbidity and mortality that minority youth experience after detention.[38]

Although the Northwestern Juvenile Project captures the proportions of psychiatric disorders within several racial and ethnic groups in the juvenile justice population,[39] it would be critical to know the relative rate of mental illness by race or ethnicity in the juvenile justice population, by comparing the proportion of psychiatric disorders within each racial or ethnic group in the juvenile justice population with the proportion of psychiatric disorders within their respective groups in the general population. The Northwestern Juvenile Project found that the sociodemographic risk factors associated with waiver to adult criminal court coincide with the sociodemographic risk factors associated with low access to mental health care, independent of need.[33] This finding suggests that the intersection between sociodemographic factors, including race and ethnicity, and poor access to mental health care for those youth with psychiatric disorders may interact with judicial discretion to increase DMC. Because race and mental health problems are both associated with juvenile justice involvement, the concern over DMC is also a concern over disparities in health care.[33] Another study found that rates of psychiatric disorders, including substance abuse disorders, and educational challenges, positively correlated with rates of recidivism.[34] Therefore, improving access to mental health care, particularly for at-risk youth, is an important consideration in reducing DMC.[36]

Family and community factors

Socioeconomic status also plays a critical role in disproportionate minority representation.[21] In 2000, 32% of African American youth lived below the poverty level.[1] Although there are no studies directly linking poverty to delinquency, poverty is linked to other risk factors for antisocial behavior, such as poor health, homelessness, and school failure.[6] Youth from low-income families may also lack parental guidance and supervision because parents may need to work more to provide for their families. Judicial personnel may base decisions on family structure and the availability of parental supervision.[21]

Institutional factors

Zero tolerance policies in school disproportionately affect the most vulnerable students: those students with multiple risk factors of psychosocial adversity, such as poverty, racial segregation, welfare, unemployment, and community violence. Further, suspension and expulsion have negative psychosocial sequelae, including decreases in socioemotional functioning, related to stigmatization from peers, avoidance and social withdrawal from school staff, and impaired academic performance.[26,40] Thus, in many cases, the punitive disciplinary style of suspension and expulsions stemming from zero tolerance results in more harm than good.

IMPLICATIONS

DMC has implications at every stage of the juvenile justice process. Unnecessary referrals to the juvenile court may not be reversible[15]; resources spent on such

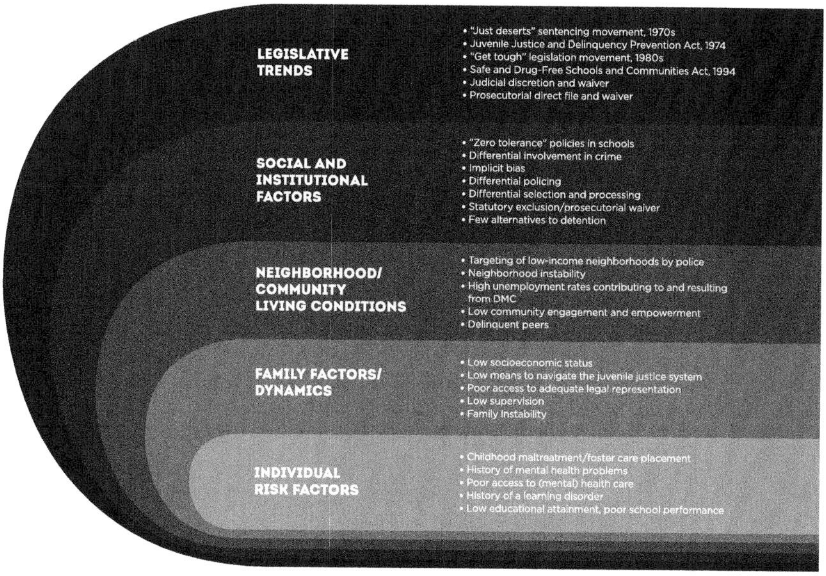

Fig. 6. Ecological framework for contextualizing and conceptualizing delinquency and DMC.

Table 2
Resources pertaining to DMC

Resource	Web site
Office of Juvenile Justice and Delinquency Prevention • Publications, programs, funding opportunities, events, statistics, and other resources	ojjdp.gov
National Disproportionate Minority Databook • Counts, rates, and relative rate indices associated with processing of delinquency cases at various decision points within the juvenile justice system	ojjdp.gov/ojstatbb/dmcdb
The Annie E. Casey Foundation • Juvenile justice reform agenda • Resources, including the Juvenile Detention Alternatives Institute • Interactive state and national data (KIDS COUNT)	aecf.org
Center for Children's Law and Policy • Resources related to key issues in juvenile justice reform, including descriptions of several current and completed projects, such as Building Blocks for Youth	cclp.org
Coalition for Juvenile Justice • Tenets to improve outcomes for youth • Description of programs, including Models for Change • Annual reports to Congress, including A Delicate Balance • Resource library	juvjustice.org
Community Justice Network for Youth • Sample curricula; eg, of how youth are processed through the juvenile justice system • Information on national and regional conferences, peer-to-peer exchanges, technical assistance, and task forces	communityjusticenetworkforyouth.org
W. Haywood Burns Institute • Interactive state data maps, publications • Description of services, including Intensive Site Engagement, Readiness Assessment Consultations, and training	burnsinstitute.org

Juvenile Justice Resource Hub • Comprehensive source of key issues, resources, reform trends, and experts in several areas of juvenile justice reform • Partnership between the National Juvenile Justice Network, the MacArthur Foundation, and the Juvenile Justice Information Exchange	jjie.org/hub
Models for Change (John D. and Catherine T. MacArthur Foundation) • Description of several areas of juvenile justice reform, including DMC • Details about annual conference • Publications and resource centers related to mental health needs, public defense for indigent youth, status offenses, and dual status youth	modelsforchange.net
National Juvenile Justice Network • Principles of reform, resources by state, publications, teleconferences, webinars • Details about annual forum	njjn.org
The Sentencing Project • Fact sheets, publications, and news in several criminal justice reform areas, including juvenile justice reform • Race and Justice Clearinghouse:>500 publications related to racial disparities in the criminal justice system	sentencingproject.org

referrals could be better spent reducing DMC. Further, detention disrupts youths' supportive family relationships as well as their educations.[18,24] Detained youth are less likely to receive a high school diploma,[2] which, in turn, increases their risk of recidivism.[25] Detention is often psychologically stressful and may exacerbate psychiatric disorders.[18] Because of DMC, minority youth likely experience these ramifications more frequently.

The Office for Juvenile Justice and Delinquency Prevention and the Centers for Disease Control and Prevention performed literature reviews and concluded that being waived to adult criminal court increases the risk of recidivism.[18] In one study, African American youth transferred to adult criminal court were more likely to be rearrested than white youth.[18] Further, automatic waivers preclude consideration of mental health problems in decisions regarding transfer.[33]

In addition to worsening outcomes for youth, DMC also affects communities in a disproportionate manner. After out-of-home placement, it is more difficult to obtain and sustain long-term employment.[5,24] The absence of the youth from the home also affects the stability of the family and the quality of life in communities.[5] Because social inequities contribute significantly to DMC, and involvement in the juvenile justice system worsens these social inequities, minority youth, their families, and communities may fare progressively worse in multiple domains.[24] However, although the JJDP Act offers financial incentives for complying with the requirement to address the causes of DMC, there are no substantial consequences if states choose not to comply.[6]

INTERVENTIONS

It is helpful to consider a social ecological model of causes of DMC, given the overlap in many of the theories discussed earlier. Such a model encompasses the dynamics and relationships between personal, social, and environmental variables. The social ecological model also provides a good vantage point from which states may develop interventions to reduce DMC (**Fig. 6**).

Several studies have outlined categories of interventions for reducing DMC. These categories include data review, cultural competency training, risk assessment instruments, community-based prevention and intervention programs, family involvement, community engagement and legislation of system-level change.[2,18,41]

Implicit bias, the preference for a group based on unconsciously held stereotypes,[24] likely affects decision making at every stage of the juvenile justice system. States may counter implicit bias by providing interagency cultural competency training[42] to law enforcement and judicial personnel through mindful awareness and education[42] on the problem of DMC. In Multnomah County, Oregon, new police officers undergo cultural competency training before they encounter youth in the community in order to increase their consciousness about DMC.[41] On a systems level, juvenile justice systems could work to reduce the case load of decision makers, examine cues in the environment that may perpetuate stereotypes, and create external checks and balances.[42]

Risk assessment instruments may perpetuate racial bias also.[41] Juvenile justice systems can create race-neutral risk assessment instruments to minimize subjectivity and bias in decisions about the appropriate level of supervision after a youth is referred to court.[18,41] Several jurisdictions have replaced ethnically biased criteria on risk assessments and created protocols to standardize detention decisions.[41]

Alternatives to juvenile detention are designed to meet the needs of youth while keeping them in the community; such interventions provide greater benefits than detention for all youth. Most alternatives incorporate 1 or more elements of house arrest, structured day or evening programs, and youth shelters.[41] Jurisdictions should also create alternatives to out-of-home placement on disposition.[2] Involving families and providers in service coordination, including connection with mental health services, reduces recidivism.[25]

States could design and implement interventions in early childhood programs to target rates of maltreatment and delinquency.[43] Community-based and school-based programs for high-risk youth can strengthen protective factors, which may reduce DMC.[6,36] For example, for African American youth, engagement with religious institutions reduces involvement in serious crime.[6] In addition, schools can minimize or eliminate zero tolerance policies in favor of reintegration and rehabilitation.[15]

Future research in the area of DMC should focus on fine-tuning the causes of this problem and examine involvement in crime by multiple ethnic groups over the life course. Specifically, because of lack of systematic documentation of ethnicity (in addition to race), studies have not examined factors of DMC for Hispanic and Latino populations to a large extent.[44] Future interventions should address differential involvement and associations with psychosocial factors in addition to differential treatment on contact with law enforcement and throughout the juvenile justice process.

RESOURCES

Table 2 provides an overview of resources pertaining to DMC.

REFERENCES

1. Sickmund M, Sladky A, Kang W. Easy access to juvenile court statistics: 1985-2013. [Online]. Available at: http://www.ojjdp.gov/ojstatbb/ezajcs/. Accessed June 27, 2015.
2. Coalition for Juvenile Justice. Disproportionate minority contact facts and resources. 2010. Available at: http://www.juvjustice.org/sites/default/files/resource-files/Disproportionate Minority Contact Fact Sheet.pdf. Accessed May 26, 2015.
3. Bishop DM, Leiber MJ, Johnson JD. Contexts of decision making in the juvenile justice system: an organizational approach to understanding minority overrepresentation. Youth Violence Juv Justice 2010;8:213–33.
4. Armour J, Hammond S. Minority youth in the juvenile justice system: disproportionate minority contact. Washington, DC: National Conference of State Legislatures; 2009.
5. Piquero AR. Disproportionate minority contact. Future Child 2008;18:59–79.
6. Rozie-Battle JL. African American teens and the neo-juvenile justice system. J Health Soc Policy 2002;15:69–79.
7. *Kent v United States*, 383 US 541, 1966.
8. *In re Gault*, 387 US 1, 1967.
9. Feld BC. Race, youth violence and the changing jurisprudence of waiver. Behav Sci Law 2001;19:3–22.
10. Bilchik S. Juvenile justice reform initiatives in the states, 1994-1996. Washington, DC: US Department of Justice, Office of Juvenile Justice and Delinquency Prevention; 1997.
11. Juvenile Justice and Delinquency Prevention Act, 42 USC § 5601, 1974.
12. Coleman AR. A disproportionate minority contact chronology: 1988 to date. US Department of Justice Office of Juvenile Justice and Delinquency Prevention.

Available at: http://www.ojjdp.gov/dmc/chronology.html. Accessed May 5, 2015.
13. Adams B, Puzzanchera C. Juvenile justice system: a national snapshot. Pittsburgh (PA): National Center for Juvenile Justice; 2007.
14. The National Coalition of State Juvenile Justice Advisory Groups. A Report on the Delicate Balance. Washington, DC: Coalition for Juvenile Justice; 1989.
15. Cobb H. Separate and unequal: disparate impact of school-based referrals to juvenile court. Harv Civ Rights-Civil Lib Law Rev 2009;44:581–95.
16. Fenning P, Rose J. Overrepresentation of African American students in exclusionary discipline: the role of school policy. Urban Educ 2007;42:536–59.
17. Casella R. Zero tolerance policy in schools: rationale, consequences, and alternatives. Teach Coll Rec 2003;105:872–92.
18. Soler M. Missed opportunity: waiver, race, data, and policy reform. La Law Rev 2010;71:17–33.
19. Hoytt EH, Schiraldi V, Smith B, et al. Pathways to juvenile detention reform: reducing racial disparities in juvenile detention. Baltimore (MD): The Annie E. Casey Foundation; 2001.
20. Gavazzi SM, Yarcheck CM, Lim J-Y. Ethnicity, gender, and global risk indicators in the lives of status offenders coming to the attention of the juvenile court. Int J Offender Ther Comp Criminol 2005;49:696–710.
21. Kakar S. Understanding the causes of disproportionate minority contact: results of focus group discussions. J Crim Justice 2006;34:369–81.
22. Pope CE, Feyerherm W. Minority status and juvenile justice processing. Crim Justice Abstr 1990;22:327–36.
23. Nicholson-Crotty S, Birchmeier Z, Valentine D. Exploring the impact of school discipline on racial disproportion in the juvenile justice system. Soc Sci Q 2009;90:1003–18.
24. Nellis A, Richardson B. Getting beyond failure: promising approaches for reducing DMC. Youth Violence and Juvenile Justice 2010;8:266–76.
25. Maschi T, Hatcher SS, Schwalbe CS, et al. Mapping the social service pathways of youth to and through the juvenile justice system: a comprehensive review. Child Youth Serv Rev 2008;30:1376–85.
26. Costenbader V, Markson S. School suspension: a study with secondary school students. J Sch Psychol 1998;36:59–82.
27. The Sentencing Project. The facts about dangers of added police in schools. 2013. Available at: http://sentencingproject.org/doc/publications/jj_Police in Schools Fact Sheet.pdf. Accessed June 26, 2015.
28. Poe-Yamagata E, Jones MA. And justice for some. Davis (CA): National Council on Crime and Delinquency; 2000.
29. Juszkiewicz J. Youth crime/adult time: is it justice served? Washington, DC: Building Blocks for Youth; 2000.
30. Arya N, Augarten I. Critical condition: African-American youth in the criminal justice system. Washington, DC: Campaign for Youth Justice; 2008.
31. Janku AD, Jiahui Y. Exploring patterns of court-ordered mental health services for juvenile offenders: is there evidence of systemic bias? Crim Justice Behav 2009; 36:402–19.
32. Teplin LA, Abram KM, McClelland GM, et al. Psychiatric disorders in youth in juvenile detention. Arch Gen Psychiatry 2002;59:1133–43.
33. Washburn JJ, Teplin LA, Voss LS, et al. Psychiatric disorders among detained youths: a comparison of youths processed in juvenile court and adult criminal court. Psychiatr Serv 2008;59:965–73.

34. Dembo R, Schmeidler J, Sue CC, et al. Psychosocial, substance use, and delinquency differences among Anglo, Hispanic white and African-American male youths entering a juvenile assessment center. Subst Use Misuse 1998;33: 1481–510.
35. Teplin LA, Welty LJ, Abram KM, et al. Prevalence and persistence of psychiatric disorders in youth after detention. Arch Gen Psychiatry 2012;69:1031–43.
36. Chapman JF, Desai RA, Falzer PR, et al. Violence risk and race in a sample of youth in juvenile detention: the potential to reduce disproportionate minority confinement. Youth Violence and Juvenile Justice 2006;4:170–84.
37. Guthrie BJ, Cooper SM, Brown C, et al. Degrees of difference among minority female juvenile offenders' psychological functioning, risk behavior engagement, and health status: a latent profile investigation. J Health Care Poor Underserved 2012;23:204–25.
38. Teplin LA, Abram KM, Washburn JJ, et al. The Northwestern Juvenile Project: overview. OJJDP juvenile justice bulletin. Washington, DC: US Department of Justice, Office of Juvenile Justice and Delinquency Prevention; 2013.
39. Teplin LA, Abram KM, McClelland GM, et al. Psychiatric disorders of youth in detention. In: Kessler CL, Kraus LJ, editors. The mental health needs of young offenders: forging paths toward reintegration and rehabilitation. New York: Cambridge University Press; 2007. p. 7–47.
40. Stinchcomb JB, Bazemore G, Riestenberg N. Beyond zero tolerance: restoring justice in secondary schools. Youth Violence Juv Justice 2006;4:123–47.
41. Cabaniss ER, Frabutt JM, Kendrick MH, et al. Reducing disproportionate minority contact in the juvenile justice system: promising practices. Aggress Violent Behav 2007;12:393–401.
42. Marsh SC. The lens of implicit bias. Juvenile and Family Justice Today 2009;16.
43. Mersky JP, Reynolds AJ. Child maltreatment and violent delinquency: disentangling main effects and subgroup effects. Child Maltreat 2007;12:246–58.
44. Kempf-Leonard K. Minority youths and juvenile justice: disproportionate minority contact after nearly 20 yrs of reform efforts. Youth Violence Juv Justice 2007;5: 71–87.

Civil and Constitutional Rights of Adjudicated Youth

Jacqueline Landess, MD, JD*

KEYWORDS

- Juvenile due process rights • Status offenders • Juvenile court

KEY POINTS

- The juvenile court has evolved since its inception to recognize greater protections and due process rights for juvenile offenders.
- Gaps or gray areas still remain, particularly in the case of status offenders and for those in preadjudicatory phases.
- Juveniles often waive fundamental rights, such as a right to counsel, likely because of a combination of factors.
- Clinicians working with youth involved with the juvenile justice system should consult their state's juvenile code to determine the specific guarantees afforded to their patients, given the significant variability from state to state in court structure, sentencing, waivers, and procedural rights.

Mental health clinicians serving child and adolescent patients are frequently asked to evaluate youth who have been arrested for various offenses or who are otherwise involved with the juvenile justice system. To help orient clinicians and other stakeholders involved with such cases, this article summarizes the history and current status of the civil and constitutional rights of youth involved in the adjudicatory process.

EARLY HISTORY OF JUVENILE JUSTICE

In 1899, Judge Richard Tuthill heard the nation's first juvenile court case in Chicago, Illinois.[1] The creation of a juvenile court was a culmination of decades-long efforts of social reformers who believed that juvenile offenders should be treated and assessed differently than adult criminals. However, the recognition that children were developmentally distinct from their adult counterparts was a fairly new concept within American society.

Disclosure Statement: The author has nothing to disclose.
University of Colorado, Aurora, CO, USA
* Forensic Psychiatry, Office of Behavioral Health, 3520 West Oxford Avenue, Denver, CO 80236.
E-mail address: Jacqueline-landess@fsm.northwestern.edu

Child Adolesc Psychiatric Clin N Am 25 (2016) 19–26
http://dx.doi.org/10.1016/j.chc.2015.08.004 **childpsych.theclinics.com**

The Evolution of the Concept of Childhood and Adolescence

Throughout Medieval times, children were treated with relative indifference. Aries,[2] in his seminal work *Centuries of Childhood*, described how children were mixed with adults soon after they were weaned, usually around the age of 7. The idea that children had specific and unique developmental needs, and were not simply miniature adults, began to develop during the Renaissance. During this time period, "the family ceased to be simply an institution for the transmission of a name and an estate—it assumed a moral and spiritual function, it moulded bodies and souls."[2]

Society's view of children as "vulnerable, innocent, passive and dependent beings who need extended preparation for life,"[3] largely evolved during the Progressive Era. This period, spanning from the 1890s to 1920s, was a time of expansive social activism and political reform within the United States; many citizens truly believed that the government "empowered by scientific expertise and the political will could attack and solve any social, economic, or political challenge the country might face."[4]

From this climate, the child-saving movement was borne. The child-savers were a "loose collection of women...from middle- and upper-class backgrounds who exercised considerable influence in...how government dealt with dependent, neglected and delinquent children."[5] These activists noted that only minimal resources existed for children who were delinquent, poor, or vagrant. No separate court or social agency existed to adjudicate and serve the needs of these youth. Despite the creation of houses of refuge (institutions for abandoned, incorrigible, or delinquent youth) in the early nineteenth century, by the late 1900s many of these institutions had been shuttered because of issues with overcrowding, staff abuse, and poor living conditions.[6]

The lack of a separate penal system for children proved especially problematic. Children as young as 7 years old were convicted for crimes, such as petty theft, and placed into jails or prisons alongside adult offenders.[7] Children younger than 7 usually were not prosecuted because of the common law defense of infancy: an "infant" could not form the prerequisite *mens rea*, or criminal intent, to commit a crime.[8] The child-savers advocated for a separate governmental system or entity in which to assess, treat, and house predelinquent, delinquent, and abandoned youth. A collaborative effort between the Chicago Women's Club (a child-saving organization), the Chicago Bar Association, and the Illinois Conference of Charities led to the creation of the nation's first juvenile court.[5]

THE CREATION OF THE JUVENILE COURT

Although Illinois was the first state to implement a juvenile court, by 1935 nearly all states had some form of a juvenile court system. The juvenile court system differed from the adult system in that (1) it was rehabilitative rather than punitive, (2) records were confidential, (3) juveniles were not placed with adult criminals, and (4) the juvenile system allowed for informal court procedures.[1]

These courts were considered civil rather than criminal courts. Thus, terminology differed within the juvenile system: for example, rather than a "verdict" being rendered, juvenile courts rendered an "adjudication" and a juvenile is found "delinquent" rather than "guilty." However, many courts, as a practical matter, interchange terminology with the adult criminal system. Due process rights may differ depending on the stage of the adjudicatory process; for instance, preliminary or dispositional hearings may have different rules than adjudicatory hearings and youth may have more limited rights while in preadjudication detention.

In addition to delinquency cases, the courts often hear dependency cases involving neglect or abuse and cases involving status offenses. It is crucial to note that there is wide variability in the structure and organization of juvenile courts from state to state; in addition, some courts have specialized courts, such as family, mental health, or drug courts, that hear juvenile cases or work in conjunction with the juvenile court.

The Doctrine of Parens Patriae and the Rehabilitative Ideal

The juvenile court's stated focus on rehabilitation rather than punishment allowed lax and informal court procedures. The philosophy underlying this approach was that strict rules of evidence were not needed given the supposed nonadversarial approach to proceedings. The court's wide latitude in determining delinquent status, adjudication, and appropriate disposition was an extension of the English doctrine of *parens patriae*, which means "parent of the country."[9] *Parens patriae* is the belief that the state has the responsibility of caring for those who cannot care for themselves. Within the juvenile court system, the state becomes a surrogate parent for adjudicated youth when parents are deemed incapable or unavailable to do so. This approach encourages a rehabilitative ideal with less formal court procedures, instead focusing on the best interests of the child. The focus was not so much on what the child did, but who the child was, and the courts were to ascertain the truth of what brought the child into the system, rather than adhering to strict rules of evidence.[7] Judge Julian Mack,[10] in *The Juvenile Court*, reflected this philosophy:

> *Why is it not just and proper to treat these juvenile offenders as we deal with the neglected children, as a wise and merciful father handles his own child whose errors are not discovered by the authorities? Why is it not the duty of the State, instead of asking merely whether a boy or a girl has committed the specific offense, to find out what he is, physically, mentally, morally, and then if it learns that he is treading the path that leads to criminality, to take him in charge, not so much to punish as to reform, not to degrade but to uplift, not to crush but to develop, not to make him a criminal but a worthy citizen.*

This reliance on a judge's subjective assessment of a child's needs, rather than the nature of the crime, seemed to be a just and admirable approach, in line with the stated rehabilitative ideal of the courts. However, this approach led to adjudicative dispositions that were inconsistent and unpredictable. For example, a youth who committed the crime of petty theft might be placed on probation or perhaps sent to a reform school, depending on the subjective assessment of his or her needs, which were inevitably influenced by an individual judge's perception and beliefs. In addition, juveniles received little to no due process protections before and during adjudicative proceedings, providing them with few safeguards against unfair outcomes. By the 1960s, it seemed that juvenile courts were shifting to a more punitive, rather than rehabilitative, model. A series of Supreme Court cases responded to this growing pattern.

THE WORST OF BOTH WORLDS: ESTABLISHMENT OF MINIMUM DUE PROCESS RIGHTS FOR JUVENILES

Beginning in the 1960s, the Supreme Court established minimum due process rights for juveniles who were accused of delinquent acts or in police custody. In 1966, the first in a trio of Supreme Court decisions was handed down that established minimum due process rights for juveniles and limited the reach of *parens patriae*. *Kent v United States* determined that juveniles facing transfer to adult court (also known as a judicial waiver proceeding) are entitled to basic due process rights, such as a hearing, effective assistance of counsel, and a "statement of reasons."[11] The Court determined that *parens patriae* was "not an invitation for procedural arbitrariness."[11] The Court famously noted that "the child receives the worst of both worlds: that he gets neither the protections accorded to adults nor the solicitous care and regenerative treatment postulated for children."[11]

Juvenile due process rights were further strengthened the following year when the Supreme Court decided the case of *In re Gault*. This was a landmark case in juvenile rights, although perhaps the victory was a symbolic one, given the lack of uniform implementation.[12] Gerald Gault was a 15-year-old youth on probation, who was charged with making an obscene telephone call to a neighbor. Gault was arrested and his parents were not notified of his arrest. Neither he nor his parents received a copy of the petition filed against him, and the alleged victim did not appear in court. Several hearings occurred, and ultimately the judge committed Gault to 6 years of juvenile detention. A similar crime, if committed by an adult, would warrant a maximum sentence of a $50 fine and 2 months in jail.[13] The Supreme Court determined that juveniles facing adjudication of delinquency and incarceration were entitled to certain due process rights under the Sixth and Fourteenth Amendments. The Court opined: "neither the Fourteenth Amendment or the Bill of Rights is for adults alone."[13] The Court determined that juveniles facing incarceration had the (1) right to confront witnesses, (2) right against self-incrimination, (3) right to counsel, and (4) right to timely notification of charges.

The case of *In re Winship* followed in 1970. Samuel Winship was a 12-year-old boy who was accused of delinquency after stealing money from a woman's pocketbook. If Winship had been an adult, this would have constituted the crime of larceny. Winship was ultimately adjudicated delinquent and committed to a training school. The lower court used the standard of preponderance of evidence in Winship's adjudicatory hearing, a lower burden of proof than the "beyond a reasonable doubt" standard used in adult criminal proceedings. The Supreme Court held that Winship's constitutional rights had been violated; in adjudicatory proceedings where a youth faces charges that would constitute a crime if he or she were an adult, the judge must abide by the "beyond a reasonable doubt" burden of proof.[14] Importantly, *Winship* did not address the standard of proof required in preliminary or dispositional stages of the court process, or the appropriate standard to use when evaluating status offenses.

JUVENILE RIGHTS POST-*GAULT*

The *Gault* decision sparked a "persistent debate about how to reconcile the promise of the juvenile court as a therapeutic instrument with requirements for due process."[15] *Gault* had a formidable impact on juvenile due process rights, although perhaps the change was not as pervasive as some might have hoped. For one, *Gault* addressed the rights of youth who are accused of delinquent acts, facing incarceration, and subject to adjudicatory proceedings; this allowed for interpretation of rights at other stages of the adjudicatory process or related to the type of offense (ie, status offenses as compared with delinquent acts). A flowchart of a hypothetical juvenile court process is displayed in **Fig. 1**; there are multiple preadjudicatory phases, with varying outcomes for each.

Another reality was that, despite the expansion of due process rights, often youth waived or failed to assert these rights. Arguably, youth waive or fail to assert their rights for varying reasons; research has shown that youth from disadvantaged backgrounds may feel disempowered and distrust the judicial system.[15] A youth's inexperience, lack of understanding, and perceived or actual coercion may lead him or her to waive rights; most youth waive their Miranda rights and fail to invoke their right to counsel.[16] This is particularly disturbing considering research by Grisso,[17] which showed that only 20.9% of juveniles adequately understood the four components of the Miranda warning, as compared with 42.3% of adults. These findings perhaps

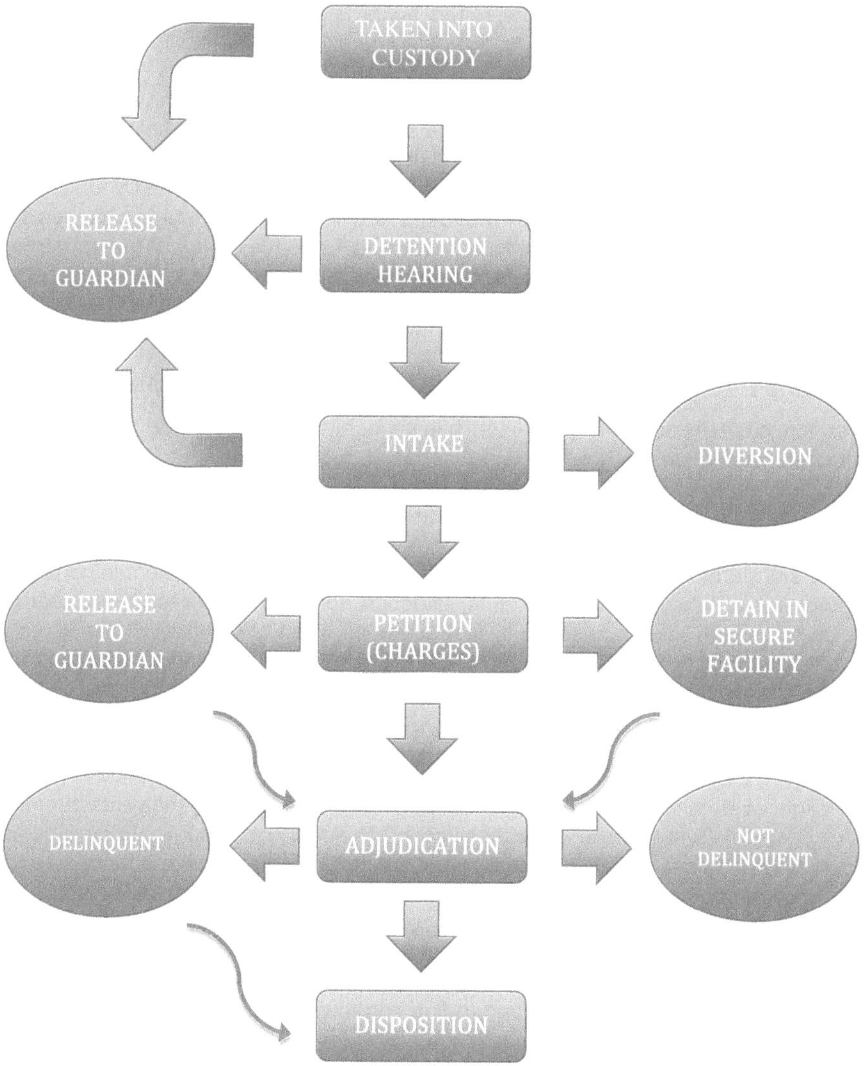

Fig. 1. Stages of the juvenile justice process: pretrial, adjudication, and postsentencing.

argue for a more assertive approach in educating and advising juvenile offenders of their rights while in custody or incarcerated.

The Juvenile Justice Delinquency Prevention Act and the Rise of the Superpredator

The 1970s saw the passage of the Juvenile Justice Delinquency Prevention Act (JJDPA), which required separation of juveniles from adult offenders, the deinstitutionalization of status offenders, and addressed disproportionate minority confinement; this legislation is further discussed later.[18] Another important shift toward increased youth autonomy (and, conceivably, greater protection of individual rights) occurred during the 1980s; the general consensus among defense attorneys evolved to recognize that juveniles were owed the same duty of loyalty as adult clients. Thus, juveniles were represented according to their expressed interests rather than the attorney determining the best interests of the child in a paternalistic way.[19]

Public sentiment toward juvenile offenders shifted in the 1980s and 1990s as the rate of juvenile crime increased.[20] Political scientist John Dilulio[21] coined the term "superpredator" to describe this new breed of juvenile offender, whom he and his colleagues went on to describe as "radically impulsive, brutally remorseless youngsters" who would only grow in numbers by the turn of the century.[22] The stage was then set for widespread public fear and panic. Fifteen years later, the theory of the superpredator has been disproved, but the media sensationalization of the superpredator led to most if not all states modifying their juvenile codes to provide for harsher sentencing and lowered the bar for waivers to adult court.[23]

Age Matters: Recent Supreme Court Decisions Regarding Juvenile Rights

Over the past decade, the pendulum has arguably begun to swing back toward increased protections for juveniles. In a series of decisions, the Supreme Court has particularly considered the impact of youth and developmental immaturity in deciding cases, such as *Roper v Simmons* (forbade death penalty for juveniles), *Graham v Florida* (no life without parole for a nonhomicide), *Miller v Alabama* (no mandatory life without parole), and *J.D.B. v North Carolina* (age is a factor in determining police custody for purpose of Miranda rights, although note that juveniles are subject to the same "totality of circumstances" test as adults when Mirandized).[24] States vary as to the availability of jury trials and the right to bail or bond, given no established precedent.[25] These rights do exist within the adult criminal system.

GAPS IN CONSTITUTIONAL PROTECTIONS: THE CASE OF THE STATUS OFFENDER

The plight of status offenders came to the attention of Congress in the years after the *Gault* decision. Status offenses are those acts that would not be criminal if committed by an adult, and are considered unacceptable solely because of the offender's age. Examples of common status offenses are provided in **Box 1**. Before 1974, status offenders were processed and incarcerated as delinquent offenders, without the same *Gault* protections. Recognizing that incarceration for a status offense was not rehabilitative and arguably unjust, Congress sought to incentivize states to find alternatives to incarceration of status offenders, and to find community-based or other approaches to rehabilitate these youth.

Thus, in 1974, Congress enacted the JJDPA, which established the Office of Juvenile Justice and Delinquency Prevention to support local and state efforts to prevent

Box 1
Examples of common status offenses

Truancy

Running away

Consumption or possession of alcohol

Consumption or possession of tobacco

Violating curfew

Being incorrigible or ungovernable

Note that the definitions of the status offenses listed likely vary from state to state.

delinquency and improve the juvenile justice system. One component of the Act was the deinstitutionalization of status offenders; states' compliance was contingent on receiving federal juvenile justice grant monies.[26]

States began to comply with the JJDPA requirements, but judges soon expressed frustration that deinstitutionalization of status offenders had no practical effect on reducing the recidivism rate of these offenders and allowed for limited rehabilitation. For instance, a youth who ran away might be diverted to a community program or nonsecure detention facility, but would often simply just run away again.

To address this issue, the Valid Court Order (VCO) exception was amended to the JJDPA in 1980. This allowed judges to place adjudicated status offenders in locked detention if they violated a court order. So if a youth ran away and was released back to his or her guardians with the court order of "do not run away" or "attend counseling" and violated either of these orders, that youth could be placed in secure detention. This process of converting a status offense to a delinquent act is known as "bootstrapping."[23] Bootstrapping allowed many status offenders to be institutionalized, even though the base offense was still status in nature.

Not every state allows for the VCO exception, and there has been a national movement to prohibit the VCO exception altogether, with proponents pointing to the amendment's disproportionate impact on females and minorities, and the limited usefulness of incarceration in addressing the root cause of status behaviors. Overall, the number of incarcerated status offenders has decreased dramatically compared with the 1970s. Other approaches divert status offenders away from the juvenile system altogether. The Coalition for Juvenile Justice Web site highlights Clark County in Washington as one example of an alternative approach; truant children in Clark County go before a community truancy board rather than a judge, and dispositions often include wraparound services to address the comprehensive needs of the child and family.[26]

SUMMARY

The juvenile court has evolved since its inception to recognize greater protections and due process rights for juvenile offenders. Gaps or gray areas still remain, particularly in the case of status offenders and for those in preadjudicatory phases. In addition, juveniles often waive fundamental rights, such as a right to counsel, likely because of a combination of factors. Clinicians working with youth involved with the juvenile justice system should consult their state's juvenile code to determine the specific guarantees afforded to their patients, given the significant variability from state to state in court structure, sentencing, waivers, and procedural rights.

REFERENCES

1. Slovenko R. Juvenile justice. In: Psychiatry in law/law in psychiatry. New York: Brunner-Routledge; 2002. p. 291–304.
2. Aries P. Centuries of childhood: a social history of family life. Translated by Robert Baldick. New York: Random House; 1962. p. 411–3.
3. Feld BC. The transformation of the juvenile court. Minn Law Rev 1991;75:691–4.
4. Sicius FJ. The progressive era: a reference guide. Santa Barbara (CA): ABC-CLIO, LLC; 2015.
5. Burfeind J, Bartusch Dawn J. Juvenile delinquency: an integrated approach. 1st edition. Sudberry (MA): Jones and Bartlett Publishers; 2005. p. 29–32.
6. Juvenile Justice History. Center on Juvenile and Criminal Justice. Available at: http://www.cjcj.org/education1/juvenile-justice-history.html. Accessed July 5, 2015.

7. Birckhead TR. Symposium: juvenile justice reform 2.0, vol. 20. J.L. & Pol'y; 2011. p. 15.
8. Bazelon LA. Exploding the superpredator myth: why infancy is the preadolescent's best defense in juvenile court. NYU L Rev 2000;75:159. Available at: http://www.nyulawreview.org/sites/default/files/pdf/NYULawReview-75-1-Bazelon.pdf.
9. Black's law dictionary. 8th edition. Cornell University Law School Legal Information Institute; 2004. p. 1144. Available at: https://www.law.cornell.edu/wex/parens_patriae. Accessed September 18, 2015.
10. Mack JW. The juvenile court. Harv Law Rev 1909;23:104–22.
11. *Kent v U.S.*, 383 U.S. 541, 557–63 (1966).
12. Buss E. The missed opportunity in Gault. Univ Chic Law Rev 2003;70:39.
13. *In re Gault*, 387 U.S. 1–50 (1967).
14. *In re Winship*, 397 U.S. 358 (1970).
15. Melton GB, Petrila J, Poythress NG, et al. Juvenile delinquency. In: Psychological evaluations for the courts. New York: Guilford Press; 2007. p. 468–70.
16. Bishop DM, Farber HB. The promise of in re Gault: promoting and protecting the right to counsel in juvenile court. Rutgers Law Rev 2007;60(125):161–8.
17. Grisso T. Juveniles' capacities to waive Miranda rights: an empirical analysis. Calif Law Rev 1980;68:1134–53.
18. Juvenile Justice and Delinquency Prevention Act (Pub. L. No. 93–415, 42 U.S.C. § 5601 et seq).
19. Sterling R. Role of Juvenile defense counsel in delinquency court. National Juvenile Defender Center; 2009. Available at: http://njdc.info/wpcontent/uploads/2013/09/NationalJuvenileDefenseStandards2013.pdf. Accessed July 27, 2015.
20. Feld BC. Violent youth and public policy: a case study of juvenile justice law reform. Minn Law Rev 1995;79:965–1022.
21. DiLulio J. The coming of the super-predators. Wkly Standard 1995;1(11):23. Available at: http://www.weeklystandard.com/Content/Protected/Articles/000/000/007/011vsbrv.asp.
22. Bennett WJ, Dilulio J, Walters J. Body count: moral poverty and how to win America's war against crime and drugs. Simon and Schuster; 1996. p. 27.
23. Scott ES. The legal construction of adolescence. Hofstra Law Rev 2000;29:547–98.
24. *Roper v Simmons*, 543 U.S. 551 (2005); *Graham v Florida*, 130 S. Ct. 2011 (2010); *Miller v Alabama*, 132 S. Ct. 2455 (2012); *J.D.B. v North Carolina*, 131 S. Ct. 2394 (2011).
25. *McKeiver v Pennsylvania*, 403 U.S. 528 (1971).
26. Deinstitutionalization of Status Offenders (DSO) Facts and Resources. Coalition for Juvenile Justice. Available at: http://sph.lsuhsc.edu/Websites/lsupublichealth/images/pdf/iphj/SOLibrary3.pdf. Accessed July 27, 2015.

Mental Health Screening and Assessment of Detained Youth

Matthew Soulier, MD[a,*], Anne McBride, MD[b]

KEYWORDS

- Juvenile justice • Screening • Assessment
- The Massachusetts Youth Screening Instrument–Version 2 • Delinquency
- Rehabilitation

KEY POINTS

- Because of the unique vulnerabilities and challenges of delinquent youth, society in association with mental health professionals has invested in the rehabilitation of juveniles.
- Effective rehabilitation begins with screening of all juveniles as close to entry into the juvenile system as possible.
- This screening should consider a structured instrument to identify those youth who need more assessment.
- Assessment of juveniles should fully explore the mental health, emotional, developmental, and social challenges confronting the youth.

JUVENILE REHABILITATION

The point of entry for a juvenile into the delinquency system has long served as a place of interest for child psychiatrists. From the early child guidance clinics that formed in Chicago in 1899[1] to the 57,190 offenders housed in juvenile facilities in 2012,[2] the arrest and detention of a juvenile signifies a breakdown in order, societal norms, and parental expectations. Although justice expects some form of punishment, this vulnerable point has also been seen as a place of opportunity to help and rehabilitate minors who commit even severe crimes. In association with mental health professionals, society has long committed resources to ensuring as many of these youth as possible are given a chance at rehabilitation.

The authors have nothing to disclose.
[a] Division of the Psychiatry and Law, University of California Davis Medical Center, 2230 Stockton Boulevard, Sacramento, CA 95817, USA; [b] Department of Psychiatry and Behavioral Sciences, University of California Davis Medical Center, 2230 Stockton Boulevard, Sacramento, CA 95817, USA
* Corresponding author.
E-mail address: mfsoulier@ucdavis.edu

Child Adolesc Psychiatric Clin N Am 25 (2016) 27–39
http://dx.doi.org/10.1016/j.chc.2015.08.002
childpsych.theclinics.com
1056-4993/16/$ – see front matter

Social reformers in the 1800s did not believe abused, neglected, and delinquent youth simply merited punishment as adults. Rather, they envisioned an opportunity to rehabilitate these youth within the delinquency system, consistent with the parens patriae doctrine, with the state functioning in a parental role. Rehabilitation toward better functioning adults could only occur if the needs and psychopathology of the delinquents were understood. Child guidance clinics were formed as a part of the juvenile courts in the early 1900s to assess the needs of these juveniles.[1]

The proper care, screening, and treatment of delinquent youth was re-emphasized throughout the 20th century as the US Supreme Court augmented juveniles' due process rights through a series of landmark cases (see Kent v United States, 1966, In re Gault, 1967).[3,4] In Estelle v Gamble (1976),[5] the US Supreme Court held that prisoners had a constitutional right to medical care, including access to care, any care that is ordered, and professional medical judgment. The Court did not specify whether the rights of Estelle extended to incarcerated youth. However, there has been substantial federal interest in the wellbeing and care of delinquent youth in the last decades.

FEDERAL RESPONSE TO JUVENILES

The Juvenile Justice and Delinquency Prevention Act was passed in 1974 and most recently authorized in 2002. This Act advocates for and establishes federal standards for the care and custody of youth in the juvenile and criminal systems. Its federal agency, the Office of Juvenile Justice and Delinquency Prevention, is dedicated to "training, technical assistance, model programs, and research and evaluation, to support state and local efforts."[6] Office of Juvenile Justice and Delinquency Prevention is a section of the United States Department of Justice. Other important oversight of detained juveniles came from the American Medial Association that began the National Commission of Correctional Health Care (NCCHC) in 1983 after studies in the 1970s confirmed that the medical care in incarcerated settings was abysmal.[7] The NCCHC has since sought to establish standards of care for incarcerated populations through publications such as the Standards for Health Services in Prisons (2014)[8] and Standards for Health Services in Juvenile Detention and Confinement Facilities (2011).[9] Mental health professionals working in delinquency settings should be at least familiar with the principles in these standards, and they may also encourage their facilities to seek voluntary accreditation with the NCCHC.

WHY INVEST IN JUVENILES?

Society invests in juvenile offenders because they are unique compared with their nondelinquent peers. The juvenile population is complex, combining prepubertal children with 20-year-olds. Chronologic age does not always match developmental age, as many youth are even more developmentally immature or intellectually impaired.[10] Crimes range from status offenses to violent felonies. Juveniles come from a variety of cultures, gang affiliations, and families. Up to 75% of juvenile offenders have one or more psychiatric diagnoses.[11] Ninety-two percent of juveniles report exposure to a major trauma.[12] There is also an overrepresentation of minority youth. Sixty-seven percent of all committed juveniles belong to a minority group, whereas they only comprise 34% of the general population.[13]

SCREENING VERSUS ASSESSMENT

Psychiatric providers are likely to encounter delinquent youth in a variety of settings, including detention centers and juvenile correctional, community, or residential

Box 1
Juvenile Screening Instruments

- MAYSI-2
- Youth Assessment & Screening Inventory (YASI)
- Global Appraisal of Individual Needs-Short Screener (GAIN-SS)
- Strengths and Difficulties Questionnaire (SDQ)

facilities. Ideally, every juvenile would be carefully and thoroughly assessed by a mental health professional at each of these sites at the time of arrival. As Grisso and colleagues[14] observe, such extensive interview of every youth is impossible. Instead, Grisso and colleagues[14] advocate for screening of every youth at admission to the juvenile justice system with the goal of identifying immediate needs, whereas assessment is performed selectively on some juveniles whose screening has signaled the need for further exploration or attention. Although screening should be completed at the point of entry, assessment can occur later with more comprehensive data. All youth entering the juvenile justice system should be screened for mental and substance use disorders, suicide and violence risk factors, and other social-emotional needs. Screening should be adequate but sensitive enough to identify youth who need more in-depth assessment within 14 days of entry according to NCCHC standards.

SCREENING INSTRUMENTS

States and juvenile facilities have adopted their own protocols to screen rather than adopting a unified approach. In a recent nationwide study[15] surveying the screening practices of facilities in all states, 24 states mandate through state statute or agency policy using a standardized screening tool during the intake process. **Box 1** lists examples of juvenile screening tools used by these states.

The Massachusetts Youth Screening Instrument–Version 2 (MAYSI-2) is the most widely used juvenile mental health screening tool (21 states reported using the MAYSI-2 in this survey).[15] It has the most empirical evidence[16–19] as an effective instrument that can be used at entry and transitional placement points in the juvenile delinquency system. The MAYSI-2 does not generate psychiatric diagnoses but rather serves to identify warning signs for further assessment.

SCREENING AND ASSESSMENT

Vignette

Darin is a 15-year-old boy who was transported to Juvenile Hall by police for his first time after he was alleged to have set a field by his house on fire. Darin's parents could not be located, although a maternal grandmother claimed to be his custodian. Darin is not currently in psychiatric treatment, but he did take methylphenidate during most of elementary school for attention-deficit/hyperactivity disorder (ADHD). Darin is sullen and not cooperative when first approached at screening. His pupils appear dilated, but he only makes scant eye contact.

Darin is typical of many juveniles entering the juvenile justice system today. He is facing a major felony crime with potentially life-altering consequences, while little is known about his actual background or the circumstance of his current care. Darin may have no experience with the juvenile system or he may have been raised in a culture or family that has had negative experiences with legal settings. Treatment providers should remember that some families and juveniles could often feel powerless or even confrontational toward a system that may limit their decision-making power and freedom. Yet, for the process of rehabilitation to begin and prevent juveniles like Darin from returning to more charges, information must be gathered in a systematic and efficient manner that balances the safety and operational demands of the facility with the assessment and treatment needs of the juvenile.

Treatment providers must be aware of their role within the larger system. Providing treatment in correctional settings can always be challenging to balance the needs for confidentiality with the sharing of information between multiple agencies such as courts and probation departments. Providers of detained youth should remember that their documentation is less likely to remain completely confidential and could be used in a manner that would not be interpreted as helpful by the juvenile if sensitive information such as admission to a crime was passed from a treatment visit to court proceedings.

Collateral sources of information should be gathered from schools, Child Protective Services (CPS), probation, past medical and psychiatric providers, and custodians. Depending on the legal status of the juvenile, a custodian will need to approve treatment decisions including the continuation of medication. **Box 2** summarizes the most essential parts of a screening and assessment of a juvenile entering the delinquency system. Although the list may not be exhaustive, these critical elements should serve as signals indicating that more in-depth assessment is needed or places that highlight where a juvenile is particularly vulnerable, neglected, or prone to future trouble.

DEVELOPMENTAL AND SOCIAL HISTORY

Juveniles should be screened and assessed for their birth history and any significant developmental or learning challenges that they have exhibited. Clinicians need to assess the custodian status and explore the juvenile's history of caretakers, if different from the current custodian. The employment and living status and parenting strengths and weaknesses of each parent should be assessed. There may be other significant attachments who should be identified and later promoted, especially in situations in which a youth is neglected. Juveniles' strengths should also be assessed. For example, what have they enjoyed? What are their hobbies and work histories? Do they have any particular social strengths? Assessment can be just as adept at identifying problems as it can be finding assets to build on and reinforce.

Current social stressors should be identified, including the effects of poverty, gang affiliation, and history of bullying (both perpetration and victimization). Furthermore, the clinician should try to ascertain why the youth has returned to juvenile detention. A prior criminal record should be obtained, and probation should detail which

Box 2
Components of Juvenile Screening and Assessment

1. Developmental and social history
2. General psychiatric history
3. Suicide risk
4. Violence risk
5. Trauma and child maltreatment
6. Substance use history
7. Special education history
8. Medical/dental
9. Sexual orientation/identity

conditions of probation were violated. Past legal experience is important, as it will not only serve as a prediction for the future, but it will also possibly identify particular vulnerabilities that invite juveniles to more risky behaviors. Prior patterns of violence and antisocial acts will guide later treatment plans.

GENERAL PSYCHIATRIC ASSESSMENT

Juveniles should be screened for the presence of a functionally impairing mental illness. Given the high rates of psychiatric illness in detained youth, facilities should screen juveniles, preferably in a structured manner, such as the MAYSI-2, with input from outside sources of information, for mental illness and the risk of violence toward themselves and others. Current outpatient psychiatric medications should be verified, and proper consent of medication should be acquired. These medications should be continued without a significant lapse in time to avoid the risk of withdrawal, decompensation in symptoms, or behavioral problems.

Individuals who screen positive or are at high risk for psychiatric conditions need a comprehensive mental health assessment by a qualified mental health professional. Assessments should include a diagnostic interview that uses the biopsychosocial model to address factors relevant to mental health. In addition to considering the other information gathered during a screening examination, assessment should include current psychiatric symptoms and detailed psychiatric history including hospitalizations, outpatient treatment, medication history, and suicidal behaviors. Collateral sources of information from past providers or current educators may refine the understanding of the juveniles.

Through the process of screening and assessment, new diagnostic considerations may arise and old diagnoses may be better updated to include new information, such as the influence of newly discovered substance use on a previously treated mood disorder. Juvenile facilities, like psychiatric facilities, can serve as important places to monitor juveniles' behaviors and patterns and improve psychiatric formulations of youth. Clinicians should balance continuing or beginning new treatment of psychiatric illness with the potential stress of legal charges and the loss of family and home that a juvenile may be experiencing.

One point of controversy can be the treatment of ADHD in juvenile facilities, especially for youth such as Darin who may have received an incorrect diagnosis but not received stimulant medication for several years. ADHD is more prevalent among detained youth and is associated with behavioral problems and a higher risk of detention in general. ADHD is not adequately discovered with the MAYSI-2 and often requires additional screening questions for adequate assessment. Those individuals at risk for ADHD should undergo a more thorough diagnostic assessment that typically includes collateral sources of information.[20] Youth with ADHD are often treated in detention facilities with medications that may include stimulants. However, misuse and noncompliance should be assessed, and clinicians and staff should be aware of the potential for misuse and diversion of ADHD medications throughout assessment and treatment.[21]

Detention facilities can always serve as potential places where gain may be sought by the false production of symptoms, otherwise known as malingering. Although the evidence is limited regarding the prevalence of malingered psychiatric symptoms in juvenile detention facilities, mental health professionals should remain vigilant to the possibility of malingering in detained youth.[22] Atypical symptoms, secondary gain, manipulative behavior, and inconsistencies between reported and observed symptoms, collateral information, or prior records, should raise concern for malingering and may warrant further assessment.

SUICIDE RISK

VIGNETTE

Mary is a 15-year-old girl entering Juvenile Hall after being charged with theft. The arresting officer alerts you that Mary had cut her wrists superficially with the handcuffs during transportation and that she reported a history of past suicide attempts. When you see Mary, she will not answer questions about suicide. How do you proceed?

Clinicians screening and assessing suicide risk in juveniles such as Mary first need an understanding of the unique risks in detained youth. Suicide was the second leading cause of death in adolescents age 10 to 18 in 2013 in the United States.[23] Detained juveniles are at an even higher risk for suicide.[24] In a study published in 2006, Gallagher and Dobrin[25] found that youth in juvenile detention facilities were almost three times more likely to die by suicide when compared to youth in the general public.[25] Suicidal ideation and past suicidal behavior are also more common in detained youth, particularly among female detainees.[11,26]

Screening for suicidal ideation and behavior is essential when entering the delinquency system. Gallagher and Dobrin[27] examined data from 3690 facilities from the 2000 Juvenile Residential Facility Census. Overall, 4.3% of facilities reported one or more juveniles who required emergency hospital care because of a suicide attempt during the previous month. The authors found that suicide screening performed on all residing juveniles within the first 24 hours after arrival was significantly linked to lower odds of serious suicide attempts and that facilities that screened only some of their youth in the 2- to 7-day period after arrival had significantly higher odds of serious suicide attempts.[27] For Mary, given her injuries, assessment would include whether she requires emergent or higher level care, which may include transfer to a more appropriate psychiatric facility.

Detained youth may not be forthcoming during evaluation. Therefore, the clinician must understand multiple risk factors that have been associated with elevated suicide risk in juvenile facilities. In a study by the National Center on Institutions and Alternatives published in 2005, Hayes[28] analyzed 79 cases of the 110 juvenile suicides that occurred in juvenile confinement facilities nationally between 1995 and 1999. Among juveniles who completed suicide, 74.3% had a history of mental illness, 53.5% were taking psychotropic medications, 73.4% had substance use history, 18.9% had medical history, 44.3% had emotional abuse history, 34.1% had physical abuse history, and 27.8% had a sexual abuse history. Regarding specific suicidal history, 69.6% had a history of suicidal behavior including suicide attempt(s), suicidal ideation or threat, or suicidal gestures or self-mutilation.[28]

In assessing suicidal ideation and behaviors among detained juveniles, Bhatta and colleagues[26] found that certain adverse life experiences including sexual abuse, homelessness, and running away from home increased the odds of suicide attempts. The authors found additional factors significantly associated with suicidal ideation and suicide attempts including female sex, physical health symptoms, having received medical care for a serious health problem in the last year, problems with alcohol abuse, problems with anger management, symptoms of depression, and a history of mental health treatment.

All detained youth should be screened and monitored for suicide risk.[22] Although suicides can occur at any time during a juvenile's detention or confinement, specific events may warrant additional vigilance for suicide risk. Juveniles should be monitored for suicide risk at initial admission into the facility; after adjudication and return to the facility; after receipt of bad news; after any type of humiliation or rejection; during confinement in isolation, segregation, or "time-out"; and after prolonged detention.[29] Moreover, youth at risk for suicide should be referred for additional evaluation by a mental health professional. **Box 3** includes components of suicide risk screening that should be included among detained youth.[22]

Box 3
Suicide risk screening components

- Past suicidal ideation or attempts
- Current ideation, threat, or plan
- Prior mental health treatment or hospitalization
- Recent significant loss (relationship, death of family member or close friend)
- History of suicidal behavior by family member or close friend
- Suicidal ideation or behavior during prior confinement
- Initiation or discontinuation of psychotropic medication(s)

Adapted from Penn JV, Thomas C. Practice parameters for the assessment and treatment of youth in juvenile detention and correctional facilities. J Am Acad Child Adolesc Psychiatry 2005;44:1085–98.

VIOLENCE RISK

Detained youth are at a higher risk for future violence and need to be screened for current and future violence risk at the time of detention and during mental health assessment. Violence risk screening and assessment are important for triaging more violent youth into secured settings and identifying dynamic risk factors that can be managed to reduce risk of future violence. Understanding the etiology and contributing factors to violent behavior is imperative for treatment planning. Although the safety and welfare of the detained youth and others must be considered, youth seclusion, isolation, and restraint should be avoided, and such violent youth require further mental health assessment. Staff training on violence prevention, treatment of violent offenders, nonphysical means of preventing or de-escalating violent behavior, proper use of medical restraint, and personal safety techniques is essential in a juvenile detention facility.[30]

Violence risk assessment includes exploring an individual's history of previous violent behavior, weapons history, exposure to violence and trauma, child maltreatment, conduct problems, substance use, psychiatric history, gang involvement, and other risk factors associated with future violence. Youth with violent histories should be referred for further assessment and treatment. Multiple standardized instruments related to violence risk have been developed. Three of the most commonly used assessments include the Structured Assessment of Violence Risk in Youth (SAVRY), the Youth Level of Service/Case Management Inventory (YLS/CMI), and the Hare Psychopathy Checklist: Youth Version.

The SAVRY is a guide for violence risk assessment in youth between ages 12 and 18 whereby the evaluator systematically reviews risk factors that have known associations to violent recidivism based on the existing scientific and professional literature.[31] The SAVRY has been found to have strong predictive validity for violent recidivism in juvenile offenders specifically, across gender and ethnicity.[32] The YLS/CMI 2.0 is a standardized instrument used to assess risk, need, and responsivity factors in male and female juvenile offenders and to formulate a case plan.[33] Bechtel and colleagues[34] and Edens and colleagues[35] studied 4482 juvenile offenders and found that the YLS/CMI predicted recidivism (receiving any type of conviction or commitment) in both juvenile institutions and community placements.[34]

The construct of juvenile psychopathy, which describes a characterologic disorder consisting of traits such as charming, glib, lacking empathy, shallow emotions, impulsive, and irresponsible, is more controversial. Some researchers maintain that labeling a youth as a psychopath is stigmatizing and misleading, as youth are still developing their identities throughout adolescence. Further, juvenile psychopathy instruments have not been found to reliably predict recidivism in adolescent girls and ethnic minorities.[35] However, a significant volume of evidence indicates that juvenile psychopathy is predictive of general and violent recidivism, and measuring psychopathy in youth can be a useful component in a broader violence risk assessment.

The Hare Psychopathy Checklist: Youth Version was adapted from the Hare Psychopathy Checklist-Revised to measure psychopathic traits in adolescents aged 12 to 18.[36] Asscher and colleagues[37] performed a meta-analysis containing 53 studies and 10,073 juvenile participants and found that psychopathy was moderately associated with delinquency, general recidivism, and violent recidivism.[37] In particular, callous-unemotional traits and impulsiveness were both strongly associated with delinquency, and impulsivity was somewhat more strongly associated with recidivism.[37]

TRAUMA AND CHILD MALTREATMENT

The frequency of exposure to trauma among detained youth is staggering. In a random sample of 898 detained youth age 10 to 18 who were part of the larger Northwestern Juvenile Project, Abram and colleagues[38] found that 92.5% of youth had experienced one or more traumas, and the mean traumatic incidents experienced was 14.6. In this study, 11.2% of the sample population met criteria for posttraumatic stress disorder within the preceding 12 months, with more than half of these individuals reporting witnessing violence as the instigating trauma.[38] Similarly, Dierkhising and colleagues[39] studied 658 adolescents within the National Child Traumatic Stress Network Core Data Set who had recent involvement in the juvenile justice system and found 90% of these adolescents reported exposure to some type of traumatic event. Of the 19 types of traumas surveyed, the most frequently experienced trauma types included loss and bereavement (61.2%), impaired caregiver (51.7%), domestic violence (51.6%), emotional abuse/psychological maltreatment (49.4%), physical maltreatment/abuse (38.6%), and community violence (34%). In this study, 23.6% of adolescents met criteria for posttraumatic stress disorder. Other significant associated problems included externalizing problems, internalizing problems, academic problems, substance/alcohol use, and concurrent child welfare involvement.[39]

Child maltreatment, in particular, is common within detained youth.[40] As defined by the Centers for Disease Control, child maltreatment is "any act or series of acts of commission or omission by a parent or other caregiver (eg, clergy, coach, teacher) that results in harm, potential for harm, or threat of harm to a child."[41] Moreover, child maltreatment is highly associated with psychiatric disorders.[40] Mental health screening in detained youth should include youth's exposure to trauma. Retrieval of CPS records is needed at the point of screening. Trauma and maltreatment exposure warrant further assessment as far as related psychiatric disorders and other adverse outcomes. Moreover, trauma-related symptoms can be misinterpreted as unwarranted psychiatric diagnoses. As mandated reporters, clinicians may be required to make appropriate referrals to CPS, particularly if learning about previously unreported child maltreatment. Further investigation into the safety of home of the custodian may be needed.

SUBSTANCE USE

Substance use is a significant and common issue in detained youth. Screening for substance use is imperative, particularly if there is concern for substance intoxication or withdrawal, which may require emergent assessment and management. The National Institute on Drug Abuse provides a chart on evidence-based screening tools for both adults and adolescents that includes links to examples of screening tools that are available at no charge (www.drugabuse.gov).[42] Valid assessment tools, such as the Alcohol Withdrawal Assessment Scoring Guidelines and the Clinical Opiate Withdrawal Scale, for alcohol/sedative and opioid withdrawal respectively, are readily available online.[43,44] If substance intoxication or recent use is suspected, urine toxicology screening may be helpful to clarify diagnoses.

For those individuals who screen positive for substance use, further assessment by a qualified health professional is warranted. Assessment should include the presence of withdrawal symptoms, substance use disorders, other substance-related disorders, and comorbid psychiatric diagnoses.[45] Youth should also be assessed for readiness to change to aid in treatment planning.[46] Youth need assessment for treatment while detained and for referral into the community.

SPECIAL EDUCATION

In 2012, 0.3% of students (approximately 17,099 youth) ages 6 through 21 received special education and related services under the Individuals with Disabilities Education Act (IDEA) in short-term detention facilities or correctional facilities.[47] In particular, those students with emotional disturbances and learning disabilities are at higher risk for arrest and detention, and these qualifying disabilities are the most common disabilities found in the juvenile justice system.[47] All newly detained youth require educational evaluations.[22] Moreover, at the time of intake, detained youth should be screened regarding previous or current involvement in special education. Screening and assessment may include collateral sources of information such as parents and guardians, prior educational records, and medical records.

Youth who are already receiving special education services under the IDEA and who have an existing Individualized Education Program (IEP) must have their IEP continued in detention or modified at the time of an IEP meeting. Most youth with disabilities who are younger than 22 years and incarcerated in adult correctional facilities are also entitled to receive services under the IDEA. During mental health and educational assessment, if a youth seems to need an initial special education evaluation or modification to existing services, referrals can be made to the appropriate school district. Referrals are typically initiated by the parent or guardian by written request, although other individuals such as educators, probation officers, or attorneys can also refer youth.[48]

MEDICAL/DENTAL

Detained youth require medical and dental[49] screening and assessment. Although a comprehensive discussion regarding full medical and dental assessment is beyond the scope of this article, several unique health care topics require special consideration in detained youth. First, youth require screening for acute medical and psychiatric problems that may warrant additional emergent evaluation and possibly transfer to an appropriate medical treatment facility. Examples of acute medical conditions include substance intoxication or withdrawal, delirium, psychosis, catatonia, or seizures.[22] Second, health professionals should be aware of the higher prevalence of sexually transmitted diseases,[50] pregnancy in girls,[51] and lack of regular primary and preventative care[52] within detained youth when performing health screenings and assessments. Third, clinicians should try to understand the influence that medical issues have on the youth's psychiatric symptoms, and vice versa.

SEXUAL ORIENTATION/IDENTITY

Mental health assessments should include age-appropriate assessments of psychosocial development for all detained youth. Clinicians should be familiar with unique developmental challenges that may be experienced by children and adolescents who are growing up gay, lesbian, bisexual, gender nonconforming, or gender discordant.[53] In particular, transgender youth, or those individuals who have a gender identity that is discordant with their anatomic sex,[53] may have specific health risks and are often at risk for physical assault and emotional abuse during detention.[54] The National Commission on Correctional Health Care has issued guidelines involving the treatment of detained transgender individuals that includes policies on health management, patient safety, and discharge planning.[54]

FUTURE DIRECTIONS

There is much to discover and explore with youth who offend to improve their rehabilitative potential. Mental health professionals should stay alert to standards and guidelines for the screening and assessment of juveniles from organizations such as the NCCHC. Screening instruments of juveniles need additional data, which will hopefully lead to further universal adaptation in more states closer to the point of entry into the delinquency system. Mental health clinicians should then work within their institutions to develop adequate assessment of the mental health needs of those youth who screen positive so that resources are invested where they are most necessary and likely to result in prosocial change.

REFERENCES

1. Weisheit RA, Alexander DM. Juvenile justice philosophy and the demise of parens patriae. In: Hancock BW, Sharp PM, editors. Criminal justice in America: theory, practice, and policy. Upper Saddle River (NJ): Prentice Hall; 1996. p. 321–32.
2. U.S. Department of Justice. Juvenile residential facility census, 2012: selected findings. Washington, DC: Office of Juvenile Justice and Delinquency Prevention. National Report Series Bulletin; 2015.
3. Kent v United States, 383 US 541 (1966).
4. In Re Gault, 387 US 1 (1967).
5. Estelle v Gamble, 429 US 97 (1976).
6. History of JJDPA. Available at: http://www.juvjustice.org/federal-policy/juvenile-justice-and-delinquency-prevention-act. Accessed May 20, 2015.
7. NCCHC Origins. Available at: http://www.ncchc.org/about. Accessed May 20, 2015.
8. National Commission on Correctional Health Care. Standards for health services in prisons. Chicago: National Commission on Correctional Health Care; 2014.
9. National Commission on Correctional Health Care. Standards for health services in juvenile detention and confinement facilities. Chicago: National Commission on Correctional Health Care; 2011.
10. U.S. Department of Justice. Psychosocial maturity and desistance from crime in a sample of serious juvenile offenders. Washington, DC: Office of Juvenile Justice and Delinquency Prevention. Juvenile Justice Bulletin; 2015.
11. Abram KM, Choe JY, Washburn JJ, et al. Suicidal ideation and behaviors among youths in juvenile detention. J Am Acad Child Adolesc Psychiatry 2008;47:291–300.

12. U.S. Department of Justice. PTSD, trauma, and comorbid psychiatric disorders in detained youth. Washington, DC: Office of Juvenile Justice and Delinquency Prevention. Juvenile Justice Bulletin; 2013.
13. Poe-Yamagata E, Jones MA. And justice for some (report). Washington, DC: National Building Blocks for Youth Initiative; 2000.
14. Grisso T, Vincent G, Seagrave D, editors. Mental health screening and assessment in juvenile justice. New York: The Guilford Press; 2005.
15. Juvenile Justice Geography, Policy, Practice & Statistics (JJGPS). Mental health screening in juvenile justice services. Pittsburgh, PA: National Center for Juvenile Justice; 2015.
16. Grisso T, Barnum R, Fletcher KE, et al. Massachusetts youth screening instrument for mental health needs of juvenile justice youths. J Am Acad Child Adolesc Psychiatry 2001;40:541–8.
17. Wasserman G, Jensen P, Ko S, et al. Mental health assessments in juvenile justice: report on the consensus conference. J Am Acad Child Adolesc Psychiatry 2003;42:751–61.
18. Cauffman E. A statewide screening of mental health symptoms among juvenile offenders in detention. J Am Acad Child Adolesc Psychiatry 2004;43:430–9.
19. Ford JD, Chapman JF, Pearson G, et al. Psychometric status and clinical utility of the MAYSI-2 with girls and boys in juvenile detention. J Psychopathol Behav Assess 2008;30:87–99.
20. Kramer J, Cox J, Kuprevich C, et al. Diagnosis and treatment of persons with attention deficit hyperactivity disorder within the jails and juvenile facilities of the United States criminal justice system: why it matters. Washington, DC: Attention Deficit Disorder Association and its ADHD Correctional Health/Justice Work Group White Paper; 2014. Available at: http://www.ncchc.org/other-resources. Accessed June 3, 2015.
21. National Commission on Correctional Health Care. Guideline for disorder management in correctional settings: adolescent attention-deficit/hyperactivity disorder. 2014. Available at: http://www.ncchc.org/resources/clinicalguides.html. Accessed June 3, 2015.
22. Penn JV, Thomas C. Practice parameters for the assessment and treatment of youth in juvenile detention and correctional facilities. J Am Acad Child Adolesc Psychiatry 2005;44:10.
23. Centers for Disease Control and Prevention. Web-based injury statistics query and reporting system (WISQARS). 2013. Available at: http://www.cdc.gov/injury/wisqars/index.html. Accessed May 19, 2015.
24. Memory JM. Juvenile suicides in secure detention facilities: correction of published rates. Death Stud 1989;13:455–63.
25. Gallagher CA, Dobrin A. Deaths in juvenile justice residential facilities. J Adolesc Health 2006;38:662–8.
26. Bhatta MP, Jefferis E, Kavadas A, et al. Suicidal behaviors among adolescents in juvenile detention: role of adverse life experiences. PLoS One 2014;9:e89408.
27. Gallagher CA, Dobrin A. The association between suicide screening practices and attempts requiring emergency care in juvenile justice facilities. J Am Acad Child Adolesc Psychiatry 2005;44:485–93.
28. Hayes LM. Juvenile suicide in confinement in the United States: results from a national survey. Crisis 2005;26:146–8.
29. Hayes LM. Guide to developing and revising suicide prevention protocols within juvenile facilities. Baltimore (MD): National Center on Institutions and Alternatives; 2011. Available at: http://www.ncianet.org. Accessed May 19, 2015.

30. National Commission on Correctional Health Care. Position statement: prevention of violence in correctional settings. 2013. Available at: http://www.ncchc.org/position-statements. Accessed May 19, 2015.
31. Borum R, Bartel P, Forth A. Structure assessment of violence risk in youth professional manual. Lutz (FL): Par; 2006.
32. Meyers JR, Schmidt F. Predictive validity of the structured assessment for violence risk in youth (SAVRY) with juvenile offenders. Crim Justice Behav 2008;35:344–55.
33. Hoge RD, Andrews DA. Youth level of service/case management inventory 2.0 user's manual. North Tonawanda (NY): Multi-Health Systems Inc; 2011.
34. Bechtel K, Lowenkamp CT, Latessa E. Assessing the risk of re-offending for juvenile offenders using the youth level of service/case management inventory. J Offender Rehabil 2007;45:85–108.
35. Edens JF, Campbell JS, Weir JM. Youth psychopathy and criminal recidivism: a meta-analysis of the psychopathy checklist measures. Law Hum Behav 2006; 31:53–75.
36. Forth AE, Kossen DS, Hare RD. Hare psychopathy checklist: youth version (PCL: YV) technical manual. North Tonawanda (NY): Multi-Health Systems Inc; 2003.
37. Asscher JJ, van Vugt ES, Stams GJ, et al. The relationship between juvenile psychopathic traits, delinquency and (violent) recidivism: a meta-analysis. J Child Psychol Psychiatry 2011;52:1134–43.
38. Abram KM, Teplin LA, Charles DR, et al. Posttraumatic stress disorder and trauma in youth in juvenile detention. Arch Gen Psychiatry 2004;61:403–10.
39. Dierkhising CB, Ko SJ, Woods-Jaeger B, et al. Trauma histories among justice-involved youth: findings from the national child traumatic stress network. Eur J Psychotraumatol 2013;4:20274.
40. King DC, Abram KM, Romero EG, et al. Childhood maltreatment and psychiatric disorders among detained youths. Psychiatr Serv 2011;62:1430–8.
41. Center for Disease Control. Child maltreatment and prevention. Injury prevention & control. 2014. Available at: http://www.cdc.gov/violenceprevention/childmaltreatment/index.html. Accessed June 3, 2015.
42. The National Institute on Drug Abuse. Available at: http://www.drugabuse.gov/nidamed-medical-health-professionals/tool-resources-your-practice/screening-assessment-drug-testing-resources/chart-evidence-based-screening-tools-adults. Accessed June 3, 2015.
43. Clinical Opiate Withdrawal Scale (COWS). Available at: http://www.drugabuse.gov/sites/default/files/files/ClinicalOpiateWithdrawalScale.pdf. Accessed June 3, 2015.
44. Sullivan JT, Sykora K, Schneiderman J, et al. Assessment of alcohol withdrawal: the revised clinical Institute withdrawal assessment for alcohol scale (CIWA-Ar). Br J Addict 1989;84:1353–7.
45. National Commission on Correctional Health Care. Position statement: substance use disorder treatment for adults and adolescents. 2010. Available at: http://www.ncchc.org/position-statements. Accessed June 3, 2015.
46. Office of Juvenile Justice and Delinquency Prevention. Underage drinking: intervention principles and practice guidelines for community corrections. 2012. Available at: www.appa-net.org/eweb/doc/appa/pubs/UDIPPGCC.pdf. Accessed June 3, 2015.
47. U.S. Department of Education, Office of Special Education and Rehabilitative Services, Office of Special Education Programs. 36th Annual Report to Congress on the Implementation of the Individuals with Disabilities Education Act, 2014. Washington, DC: U.S. Department of Education; 2014.

48. Burrell S, Warboys L. Special education and the juvenile justice system. Washington, DC: Office of Juvenile Justice and Delinquency Prevention Juvenile Justice Bulletin; 2000.
49. Adu-Tutu M, Shields TE. Guidelines for a correctional dental health care system. 2014. Available at: http://www.ncchc.org/other-resources. Accessed June 3, 2015.
50. National Commission on Correctional Health Care. Position statement: STD testing for adolescents and adults upon admission to correctional facilities. 2014. Available at: http://www.ncchc.org/position-statements. Accessed June 3, 2015.
51. Sufrin C. Pregnancy and postpartum care in correctional settings. 2014. Available at: http://www.ncchc.org/other-resources. Accessed June 3, 2015.
52. National Commission on Correctional Health Care. Position statement: health care funding for incarcerated youth. 2014. Available at: http://www.ncchc.org/position-statements. Accessed June 3, 2015.
53. Adelson SL, American Academy of Child and Adolescent Psychiatry (AACAP) Committee on Quality Issues (CQI). Practice parameter on gay, lesbian, or bisexual sexual orientation, gender nonconformity, and gender discordance in children and adolescents. J Am Acad Child Adolesc Psychiatry 2012;51:957–74.
54. National Commission on Correctional Health Care. Position statement: transgender, transsexual, and gender nonconforming health care in correctional settings. 2015. Available at: http://www.ncchc.org/position-statements. Accessed June 3, 2015.

Transfer of Juvenile Cases to Criminal Court

Soo Jung Lee, MD*, Louis J. Kraus, MD

KEYWORDS

• Juvenile court • Juvenile transfers • Waiver hearings

KEY POINTS

- Waivers for juvenile transfer to adult court follow the 1966 *Kent v. United States* US Supreme Court decision.
- Waivers can include: judicial, prosecutor discretion, and mandatory waivers.
- Waivers are typically driven by the violent nature of the offense of which the juvenile is accused. Other influential factors include proclivity for recidivism, culpability, and amenability to rehabilitation.
- In the late 1970s, there was increased skepticism in the rehabilitation model, which increased waiver proceedings in court and juvenile transfers to criminal court.
- Recent research in neurocognitive development allows one to question the construct of transferring youth to adult court, subjecting adult penalties to an individual with an underdeveloped brain.

MODERN HISTORY OF CHILDREN

Childhood, which is presently understood as the period during which a person is in ages 0 to 18 years, has been theorized to be a modern concept. In the mid-20th century, Philippe Ariès argued that the concept of childhood is a rather recent discovery, since the 17th century, and not innate to the inception of mankind. Prior to the 1600s, children above the age of 6 years were viewed as miniadults, indistinguishable from adult status.[1] For several centuries, children were seen as property, capable of contributing to family work and being of economical value, no different than a barnyard animal. This view on children has subjected them to neglect and abuse in periods of immigration, industrialization, and urbanization. As children started developing their

The authors have nothing to disclose.
Section of Child and Adolescent Psychiatry, Autism Assessment, Research, and Treatment Services [AARTS] Center, Rush University Medical Center, 1645 West Jackson Street, Suite 603, Chicago, IL 60612, USA
* Corresponding author.
E-mail address: soo_j_lee@rush.edu

Child Adolesc Psychiatric Clin N Am 25 (2016) 41–47
http://dx.doi.org/10.1016/j.chc.2015.08.011 childpsych.theclinics.com
1056-4993/16/$ – see front matter

own entity and transitioned from property to person status, their vulnerability and special needs were recognized, cultivating a societal change to care, educate, and protect children.[2] Child labor laws, protection laws, and compulsory school laws started to take force in the late 1800s.

JUVENILE COURT

In the late 19th century, the first juvenile court system in the United States was developed as a result of the Illinois Juvenile Court Act of 1899. The juvenile court system focused on rehabilitation over punishment under the parens patriae model. Other states quickly adapted to this system, and all but 2 states had juvenile courts by 1925.[3] In 1909, the first juvenile mental health service was established, the Juvenile Psychopathic Institute, with Dr, William Healy[4] in support of the rehabilitative model and scientific injury.

Prior to the development of the juvenile court system, the English common law was applied to youth offenses. Under the English common law, individuals younger than 7 years of age were considered incompetent. Children between 7 and 14 years of age were also considered incompetent unless proven otherwise by prosecutors. However, individuals older than 14 years of age were viewed as adults, and therefore accountable as such, subjecting them to the same punishment, including the death penalty.[4] At the present time, the age of culpability has been shifted upward, where children are considered incompetent whereas teenagers are generally considered not fully culpable below the age of 18 years.

The establishment of juvenile courts did not eliminate the possibility of criminal court sentencing for youth offenders. Juvenile offenders have been subject to criminal court transfers, largely at the discretion of juvenile court judges. Judicial waivers were the primary method of juvenile transfer to adult court during the last century. Despite being tried as an adult in criminal court, constitutional protection was not established for transferred youths until the second half of the 1900s. In the 1960s to 1970s, a number of US Supreme Court decisions addressed legal rights of children, with growing appreciation of punitive practices in the juvenile courts. The US Supreme Court case, *Kent v. United States* first brought attention to the compromised constitutional rights of minors in juvenile court.[5] This case recognized that youths were being transferred to criminal court through judicial waivers based on vague assessments, forfeiting the rehabilitative services inherent to the juvenile justice system, while being denied the same legal protection granted to adults in criminal courts. In another US Supreme Court case, it was determined that juveniles have the right to notification of charges, legal counsel, and other trial rights, awarding them adult criminal due process protections in criminal court.[6]

METHODS OF TRANSFER

Juvenile cases can be transferred to criminal court through 3 methods: judicial waivers, concurrent jurisdiction, and statutory exclusion. In a judicial waiver, a judge determines the transfer. The *Kent v. United States* case helped establish the discretionary judicial waiver and the transfer criteria in which individual and legal factors are taken into consideration when determining transfer to criminal court. The transfer criteria, also known as the *Kent* criteria, evaluate the offending youth's maturity, seriousness of offense, public safety, amenability, prior legal history, and response to the juvenile system. In a concurrent jurisdiction waiver, also known as prosecutor discretion waiver, the prosecutor determines to file the juvenile case in juvenile court or criminal court without judicial review based upon the type of offense committed.

Additionally, statutory exclusion laws mandate transfers from juvenile court to criminal court based on certain charges, deprived of any transfer evaluation and considerations of otherwise mitigating factors.[7]

RECENT TRENDS

In the 1980s and 1990s, there has been an upward trend in youth violence and serious crimes,[8] which has plateaued in the following decades. Meanwhile, skepticism of the rehabilitation model grew with unsuccessful rehabilitative efforts.[9] In response to societal demands for punishment, there was a punitive shift in juvenile courts. Policies were modified to further enable juvenile transfers to criminal court[10] by adding other methods of transfer other than judicial waivers. This led to a rise in juvenile transfer to criminal court between 1987 and 1996,[11] peaking in 1994 with 13,600 waived juvenile cases.[12] More youths were sentenced with harsher punishment, increasing the number of juvenile offenders sentenced to life without parole or capital punishment.

ADOLESCENT DEVELOPMENT

Adolescence is a turbulent developmental period in which youths experience a multitude of changes. Adolescents struggle with a dichotomous state of wanting independence while parental dependency continues. Adolescents have increased level of identification and interaction with peers, novelty-seeking behavior, and risky behavior. There is growing body of literature in psychosocial and neurocognitive development, which recognizes several key features salient during adolescence. It is important to consider these attributes when determining culpability of an adolescent.

Immaturity, inherent to adolescence, is a critical factor in behavior. There is immaturity in neurocognitive development and psychosocial development. Brain development continues into adulthood, with differential development in the central nervous system.[13] In neurocognitive development, the socioemotional system develops before the cognitive control system. The limbic system is a key structure for the socioemotional system, which plays a role in reward and emotional experiences. The cognitive control system is comprised of the frontal cortex and modulates executive function involved with impulse control, planning, assessment of risk and rewards, and reasoning. The temporal developmental discrepancy between the 2 systems may explain adolescents' tendency for high-risk behavior, where reward seeking overshadows the underdeveloped executive function system.[14] Adolescents are impulsive, novelty seeking, and have undeveloped ability for risk assessment and long-term planning.[14–16] The propensity for risky behavior is further enhanced by presence of peers.[17] Identification with peers and peer interaction encompass a normative process for adolescents, and adolescents are more likely to be influenced by peers compared with adults. This phenomenon is also present in the legal system, where many juvenile offenses are group occurrences, unlike adults, who often commit crimes independently.[18] Another mitigating factor is that teenagers do not have fully formed character and have malleable personality.[16,19] Pathologic personality traits found in adolescents tend to diminish with age and do not predict personality disorders in adulthood in a meaningful way.[20] Furthermore, adolescents as a group are aggressive. However, the aggressive behavior does not persist, and is a transitory phase for most youths.[21]

The developmental immaturity during adolescence has been recognized by the judicial system and has influenced recent court decisions. In *Roper v. Simmons* (2005), the US Supreme Court ruled the death penalty for capital offenses committed as a juvenile as unconstitutional.[22] This decision was made based on 3 factors mitigating juvenile culpability. First, juveniles are immature and irresponsible compared with adults. Second, juveniles are more likely to be influenced by external factors. Lastly, juvenile character is not well developed.[16,23]

There are 3 landmark cases addressing juvenile life without parole. In *Graham v. Florida*,[24] the US Supreme Court determined that juvenile life without parole for nonhomicidal offense is unconstitutional based on neurodevelopmental immaturity and underdeveloped character. In 2 cases, *Miller v. Alabama* (2012) and *Jackson v. Hobbs* (2012), the US Supreme Court held that mandatory juvenile life without parole for capital offenses was unconstitutional.[25] Since 1994, the number of cases judicially waived to criminal court has been steadily declining, with a 61% decline in 2011.[12] However, there continue to be complexities regarding state follow-through, especially with those already incarcerated for life without parole.

FORENSIC EVALUATION FOR JUVENILE TRANSFERS TO CRIMINAL COURT

After the US Supreme Court decision on *Kent v. United States* case,[5] forensic child psychiatrists utilized the transfer criteria when evaluating a juvenile for judicial waiver. The criteria were based on several pertinent legal and individual factors illuminated by the US Supreme Court. Legal considerations included the nature and severity of offense, legal history, and the youth's response to prior rehabilitation. The individual factors included the youth's amenability to treatment, maturity, and risk for future violence. The legal factors were evaluated by juvenile courts, while forensic child psychiatrists were asked to evaluate individual factors.[26] Although this provided a starting point for transfer evaluations, this consequential assessment was not based on any aggregate of evidence.

Recent literature expansions in youth development, individual factors, and environmental factors have made forensic evaluations increasingly complex. Although a clear guideline for transfer evaluations is currently unavailable, professional organizations have provided recommendations on forensic evaluations in youths given the gravity of an evaluation and recommendations. In a recent study completed in the Maryland juvenile justice system, Means and colleagues[27] found that the most influential factor in a judge's decision for juvenile transfer to criminal court was the expert's opinion.

When assessing a youth regarding a question of transfer or waiver, it is important to be as comprehensive as possible, with the evaluation completed by a specialty-trained forensic child psychiatrist or psychologist. Initially, there should be a brief interview with the consulting attorney to establish the issues at hand and additional needs to complete a comprehensive evaluation. A request from the attorney regarding collateral information should include, among other things, all available educational records, special education records if existent, all mental health records, complete delinquency history, and a parent or guardian interview. The juvenile offender must be interviewed, and the forensic psychiatrist should provide clear explanations of the purpose of the evaluation, the psychiatrist's role, and the exceptions of confidentiality in a court-ordered evaluation. The evaluator should have good understanding of the legal proceedings, policies, and current psychiatric treatment,[28] along with potential mitigating factors for culpability, risk for recidivism or future violence, and factors promoting rehabilitation. Assessing for a juvenile offender's culpability, amenability, and ultimately disposition is a complex processes. This demands further exploration and robust studies to direct forensic evaluations while professional organizations guide legislative and judicial figures.

CLINICAL VIGNETTES

Johnny is a 15-year old white boy who is a freshman attending a public high school in a large metropolitan city, where he lives with his mother and 2 older brothers. He has been recently arrested for assaulting a person and stealing a car. Because of the nature of his current offense, Johnny is being considered for transfer to criminal court, and a forensic psychiatrist has been consulted.

Johnny has a history of 3 psychiatric hospitalizations, which was unknown to the legal system at the time of arrest. Primary presenting symptoms during his hospitalizations appeared to have been for behavioral issues. However, with careful and complete review of his medical records, an expansive range of behaviors was appreciated, including taking his mother's car, driving 90 miles per hour, walking around naked in the presence of others, and not being bothered by his behavior, with a sense of entitlement.

His initial pharmacotherapy included medication for attention-deficit/hyperactivity disorder [ADHD], and by his third hospitalization, he was prescribed risperidone with strong suspicions for bipolar disorder. For every hospital readmission, Johnny was found noncompliant with his medication despite strong recommendations for follow-up with a community mental health provider. His mother reported that when she attempted to make an appointment with a psychiatrist, it was only permitted if Johnny already had an established psychotherapist within the same community mental health center. However, the community mental health centers did not have any openings for psychotherapy services, and the mother was informed that the estimated minimum wait time was 3 months. Johnny's pediatrician was unwilling to prescribe psychotropic medications, because the pediatrician was concerned about the malpractice lawsuits secondary to the adverse effect profile of these medications. Furthermore, the pediatrician had no referral options for Johnny.

After being discharged from his third inpatient psychiatric treatment, Johnny had been noncompliant with medication for 3 weeks when his mother appreciated worsening mood, agitation, and a growing suspicion for most of his family members' behavior, which was conspicuous and nonthreatening. Johnny shoved a man into the ground, took his car keys, and stole the man's car, leading to his current arrest. He was given numerous charges including battery in the process of a felony offense. The state's attorney petitioned the court to waive Johnny to adult court because of the seriousness of the crime, its violent nature, and his history of 2 prior offenses in the juvenile court system. The prior offenses were nonviolent and were all related to theft from different stores. The public defender was able to obtain funding for consultation with a forensic child psychiatrist for a transfer to criminal court evaluation. The evaluator requested all available mental health records, education records, and delinquency records from the juvenile court. It took 2 months to obtain all of the records. Some came in from subpoenas, and others with the assistance of Johnny's mother. The educational records show that Johnny had been in special education since the third grade for underlying learning disabilities and ADHD, which were categorized under other health impaired (OHI). Johnny was diagnosed with ADHD in second grade.

Johnny had been on a number of different stimulant and nonstimulant medications for ADHD symptoms, with variable responses to treatment. His learning disability was primarily in reading, although he also had low average scoring in mathematics. There were essentially no behavioral difficulties reported with Johnny until the seventh grade. However, in seventh grade, the disruptive behavior started emerging, and teachers reported occasional talking back, coming in late to class, not completing homework, and not participating well in group projects. Despite other complaints, Johnny was not getting into fights, and was not a member of a gang.

The first time Johnny's mental health records were reviewed and summarized during all of his juvenile justice system activity was during this evaluation. As previously mentioned, Johnny has had 3 hospitalizations with varying symptom presentation including ADHD symptoms, behavioral difficulties, and symptoms of mania. Inpatient notes reported that Johnny had a positive response to Risperdal. Johnny's third hospitalization was for a duration of two-and one- half weeks. During his admission, his mother and treating psychiatrist described many symptom improvements.

Johnny's mother reported that within a few days following discharge from the hospital, Johnny began missing some doses of his medication. Within a week, mother realized that he had been completely noncompliant with medication. As described, she was not able to set up a follow-up appointment for him. She reported having checked 3 different community mental health centers without the ability to make an appointment. As seeking further outside of her catchment area, she was informed that she was not qualified to go to those mental health centers because of where she lived.

Johnny was belligerent when taken into custody. He was swearing, among other things. He said he could not understand why this was being done to him and believed that he had every right to that car. Because of the seriousness of Johnny's behavior and the possibility of transfer to adult court, he was not sent home and was kept at the predetention juvenile facility in the city. At the time of the evaluation, Johnny, had already been in the facility for 2 weeks, and had not yet been seen by a psychiatrist. He had a three-quarter page initial screening evaluation completed by an advanced nurse practitioner that primarily focused on suicide risk. This evaluation stated that Johnny's current behavioral problems were diagnostic of adolescent-onset conduct disorder, and that he has a history of ADHD.

When the child psychiatrist examined Johnny, she first noted his rapid, pressured speech and that there was a hypervigilant quality to his presentation. After an extensive interview with Johnny and his mother, and obtaining collateral from other family members, the psychiatrist was able to formulate a clearer clinical picture and appreciate a history of affective disorders in first-degree relatives. The psychiatrist made a diagnosis of a bipolar disorder. There was also a likely comorbid diagnosis of ADHD, but this was less of an immediate concern. The expert witness' opinion was that Johnny could be helped if adequate treatment was put into place, within a reasonable time frame that was no longer than his juvenile sentence. Ideally, following this treatment he would be stable enough to return back home. She also felt that it would be important for Johnny to be reassessed by his school district, considered for further educational eligibility, and provided with interventions to best accommodate his educational experience.

In this testimony, the core components of the psychiatric evaluation were presented. It was the view of the juvenile court judge that there were significant factors mitigating Johnny's culpability, particularly related to Johnny's underlying mental illness. Based on this testimony, the juvenile offender's mental health conditions were reasonably expected to be helped during the time of his juvenile sentence. Furthermore, this was his first violent offense, and this offense did not result in serious injury to another person. With these considerations, the judge's decision was to not transfer Johnny to adult court.

REFERENCES

1. Ariès P. Centuries of childhood: a social history of family life. Trans. Robert Baldick. New York: Vintage; 1962.
2. Hart SN. From property to person status: historical perspective on children's rights. Am Psychol 1991;46(1):53–9.
3. Billick S, Lubit R, Rosner R, editors. Juvenile delinquency. Principles and practice of forensic psychiatry. New York: Oxford University Press; 2003.
4. Soulier MF, Scott CL. Juveniles in court. Harv Rev Psychiatry 2010;18(6):317–25.
5. Kent v. United States, 383 U.S. 541 (1966).
6. Kraus L. Standards for Juvenile Detention and Confinement Facilities, Recommendations for Juvenile Justice Reform, Monograph, October 2001.
7. Kraus LJ, Arroyo W, editors. Recommendations for juvenile justice reform, 2nd edition [monograph]. 2005. Available at: https://aacap.org. Accessed August 17, 2015.
8. Dahlberg LL. Youth violence in the United States. Major trends, risk factors, and prevention approaches. Am J Prev Med 1998;14(4):259–72.
9. Sechrest L, White SO, Brown ED. Assembly of behavioral and social sciences (U.S.). Panel on research on rehabilitative techniques. The rehabilitation of

criminal offenders: problems and prospects. Washington, DC: National Academy of Sciences; 1979.
10. Shook JJ. Looking back and thinking forward: examining the consequences of policies and practices that treat juveniles as adults. J Evid Based Soc Work 2014;11:392–403.
11. Stahl A. Delinquency cases waived to criminal court, 1987–1996. Washington, DC: US Department of Justice, Office of Justice Programs, Office of Juvenile Justice and Delinquency Prevention; 1999. Available at: https://www.ncjrs.gov. Accessed August 17, 2015.
12. Hockenberry S, Puzzanchera C. Delinquency cases waived to criminal court, 2011. Fact sheet. Washington, DC: US Department of Justice; Office of Justice Programs; Office of Juvenile Justice and Delinquency Prevention; 2014. Available at: https://www.ncjrs.gov. Accessed August 17, 2015.
13. Giedd JN. The teen brain: insights from neuroimaging. J Adolesc Health 2008; 42(4):335–43.
14. Steinberg L. A social neuroscience perspective on adolescent risk-taking. Dev Rev 2008;28(1):78–106.
15. Luna B, Padmanabhan A, O'Hearn K. What has fMRI told us about the development of cognitive control through adolescence? Brain Cogn 2010;72(1): 101–13.
16. Steinberg L, Scott ES. Less guilty by reason of adolescence: developmental immaturity, diminished responsibilities, and the juvenile death penalty. Am Psychol 2003;58(12):1009–18.
17. Gardner M, Steinburg L. Peer influence on risk taking, risk preference, and risky decision making in adolescence and adulthood: an experimental study. Dev Psychol 2005;41:625–35.
18. Zimring FE. American juvenile justice. New York: Oxford University Press; 2005.
19. Ash P. But he knew it was wrong: evaluating adolescent culpability. J Am Acad Psychiatry Law 2012;40(1):21–32.
20. Cohen P, Crawford TN, Johnson JG, et al. The children in the community study of developmental course of personality disorder. J Personal Disord 2005;19(5): 466–86.
21. Elliott DS. Serious violent offenders: onset, developmental course, and termination. The American Society of Criminology 1993 Presidential Address. Criminology 1994;32(1):1–21.
22. Roper v. Simmons, 543 U.S. 551 (2005).
23. Fabian JM. Applying Roper v. Simmons in Juvenile Transfer and Waiver Proceedings: a legal and neuroscientific inquiry. Int J Offender Ther Comp Criminol 2011; 55(5):732–55.
24. Graham v. Florida, 130 S. Ct. 2011 (2010).
25. Bath E, Pope K, Ijadi-Maghsoodi R, et al. Juvenile life without parole: updates on legislative and judicial trends and on facilitating fair sentencing. J Am Acad Child Adolesc Psychiatry 2015;54(5):343–7.
26. Kruth IP, Brodskey SL. Clinical evaluations for transfer of juveniles to criminal court: current practices and future research. Behav Sci Law 1997;15:151–65.
27. Means RF, Heller LD, Janofsky JS. Transferring juvenile defendants from adult to juvenile court: how Maryland forensic evaluators and judges reach their decisions. J Am Acad Psychiatry Law 2012;40(3):333–40.
28. Kraus LJ, Thomas CR, Bukstein OG, et al. Practice parameter for child and adolescent forensic evaluation. J Am Acad Child Adolesc Psychiatry 2011; 50(12):1299–312.

Juvenile Competency to Stand Trial

Sofia T. Stepanyan, BA[a,*], Shawn S. Sidhu, MD[b], Eraka Bath, MD[c]

KEYWORDS

- Juvenile competency to stand trial • Juvenile competency restoration
- Juvenile competency remediation • Juvenile competency assessment
- Correlates of juvenile competency to stand trial

KEY POINTS

- Juvenile competency to stand trial is part of the due process rights that are constitutionally protected and involves a defendant's ability to consult with a lawyer and understand both courtroom proceedings and the charges being filed.
- Competency evaluations are most often referred by judges or attorneys and are typically completed by psychiatrists or psychologists with forensic training or work experience.
- Mental illness, intellectual disability, developmental disorders, and developmental immaturity are the 4 main factors considered in most juvenile competency evaluations.
- Competency assessment tools can be broken down into the following 3 categories: clinical measures and assessment techniques, forensically relevant instruments, and forensic assessment instruments.
- Restoration of competence, sometimes referred to as competency remediation or attainment involves both treating underlying conditions contributing to incompetency and educating the defendant on the legal process.

Dr E. Bath is the consulting psychiatrist to the Los Angeles County Juvenile Mental Health Court and is a member of the AACAP Juvenile Justice Committee. She has received funding from the National Institutes of Health (National Institute on Minority Health And Health Disparities, Award Number P20MD000182) and the Los Angeles County Department of Probation. Dr S.S. Sidhu receives royalties from the American Psychiatric Association for his contribution to continuing medical education questions for the journal *FOCUS*. Dr S.T. Stepanyan has nothing to disclose.

[a] Developmental Psychology, Department of Psychology, University of California, Riverside, 900 University Avenue, Riverside, CA 92521, USA; [b] Department of Psychiatry, University of New Mexico, 2400 Tucker Avenue MSC 095030, Albuquerque, NM 87131, USA; [c] Child Forensic Services, Department of Psychiatry, UCLA Neuropsychiatric Institute, 300 Medical Plaza, Room 1243, Los Angeles, CA 90095, USA
* Corresponding author.
E-mail address: sstep004@ucr.edu

Child Adolesc Psychiatric Clin N Am 25 (2016) 49–59
http://dx.doi.org/10.1016/j.chc.2015.08.008 childpsych.theclinics.com

Juvenile competency to stand trial (CST) has increasingly become a subject of great significance in forensic and psychological research in recent years, being that CST is an important aspect of due process protections. The legal term "due process" protections refers to civil rights that are protected under the V and XIV Amendments of the *United States Constitution*, in order to ensure fairness and constitutionality of the legal process. The adult standard for CST was derived from an English common law and was articulated in a landmark decision[1] by the United States Supreme Court (362 US 405, 1960). According to the Dusky standard, the "test must be whether he (the defendant) has sufficient present ability to consult with his lawyer with a reasonable degree of rational understanding ... and whether he has a rational as well as factual understanding of the proceedings against him." Although CST status is not related to a defendant's culpability, it is an important aspect of the legal proceedings, because it would be a violation of a defendant's due process protections to subject him or her to legal proceedings if incompetent to stand trial. In essence, CST, although not specifically a guaranteed right, lies at the core of fair and unbiased assessment of accountability.

Juvenile CST has received increasing attention over the years and is a relatively new concept for juvenile populations, given that it was rarely applied in the juvenile courts for most of the 20th century. Because juvenile courts operated with the philosophy of providing rehabilitation instead of punishment, court proceedings were largely informal and nonadversarial, working under the assumption that the informal nature of those proceedings would align better with the rehabilitative purpose of those courts.[2] For this reason, juvenile courts were allowed to operate without the requirements for protection of due process rights offered to adults in criminal courts. However, significant challenges to the rehabilitative philosophy of the juvenile courts emerged when the US Supreme Court started to question the success of this philosophy.[3] More often placement in the juvenile facility resulted in deprivation of freedom, rather than serving a rehabilitative purpose.[3] Consequently, in *In re Gault*,[4] the Supreme Court offered many of the same due process rights to the juveniles as applied to adults in criminal courts.

There is variance among states on what the legal predicates are to issue a finding of incompetency, and for most states, a finding of incompetency to stand trial (IST) may be issued when there is the presence of a mental illness, developmental disorder, or intellectual disability that is negatively impacting a defendant's legal decision-making. In California, for instance, the Dusky standard is interpreted through Penal Code section 1367, where CST is defined as being "a result of a mental disorder or developmental disability." According to this definition, the presence of impairment in any of the above-mentioned domains is necessary but not sufficient for making decisions about IST. The issue to be determined by the courts and the forensic evaluator is to what extent existing mental disorders inhibit someone's ability to meet the Dusky requirements of rational understanding and capacity to consult with a counsel.[5] The work on CST was based on the original work of University of Virginia Law Professor Richard Bonnie, who distinguished between 2 types of competency: basic and decisional.[6] Basic legal competence refers to the fundamental knowledge and understanding of criminal charges, judicial concept and procedures, and general ability to work with defense counsel. On the other hand, decisional competence is the quality of the defendant's reasoning process, which is one of the major components of the Dusky standard.[6]

Four main factors considered in Juvenile Competency to Stand Trial (JCST) evaluations in the juvenile populations are mental illness, intellectual disability, developmental disorders, and developmental immaturity. Existence of serious mental health problems is especially important to consider in JCST evaluations, because juveniles in the correction system display similar levels of mental disabilities as adults. Some researchers have found that 66% to 75% of detained youth may be suffering from at least one psychiatric disorder, compared with only 20% in the general population.[7] Furthermore, there is also evidence to indicate that most of these detained youths may be exhibiting comorbid psychiatric conditions.[7] Although the presence of mental disorders in inmate populations makes competency determinations quite difficult for adults, these problems may become more complex for juveniles due to the wide range of symptom variability during developmental stages. As mentioned by Larson and Grisso,[8] symptoms and behaviors exhibited at one developmental stage may be exhibited differently at another stage; consequently, it is difficult to assess which behaviors will persist over time and which behaviors will turn into lifelong mental illnesses.

Intellectual disabilities are also overrepresented in juvenile delinquency population and may therefore be important predictors of the juvenile competency status. Epidemiologic studies have indicated that prevalence rates of intellectual disabilities among incarcerated youth significantly exceed the rates of the normal population. For instance, data obtained from the National Survey of State Departments of Juvenile Corrections showed that 12.6% of youth in state juvenile facilities have a primary diagnosis of mental retardation compared with 1.6% of school-aged youth in the general population. Furthermore, the same study has also demonstrated higher prevalence rates of learning disabilities among juvenile detainee populations, indicating that the rates of those disabilities reached 36% in young offenders, compared with 7% to 12% in the regular population of school-aged children.[9] These mental disorders could lead to further problems with abstract reasoning or executive functioning, thus compromising juveniles' understanding of the legal proceedings and their ability to meaningfully participate in their own defense.[8] Moreover, research has shown that many higher-order cognitive functions required for full understanding of legal proceedings are compromised in juveniles, particularly due to underdeveloped psychological, physiologic, neurologic, and cognitive intellectual systems. As a result, many adolescents, particularly those younger than 14 to 15 years of age, are not yet fully capable of meaningfully participating in their own defense.[10,11]

Currently, there is an increased need for understanding the complexities regarding determining juvenile CST status. First, legal standards about CST have been mainly focused on adult population; therefore, states need guidance in order to develop meaningful laws in the area.[11] A growing body of literature has demonstrated that most incarcerated youths exhibit mental and intellectual deficits similar to those seen in the adult population; consequently, it is absolutely crucial that mental disorders and intellectual disability be weighted heavily in the evaluations of adjudicative competence. Moreover, mental health professionals performing competency evaluations on adolescences need guidance in understanding the effects of developmental status for assessing deficits in the legally relevant abilities.[11] Juvenile CST evaluations could also help identify the vulnerable youth, who might not otherwise have the opportunity to receive any mental health treatment. A large number of young offenders with a wide range of mental disorders and intellectual disabilities receive mental health treatment only after their first contact with law enforcement. More specifically, most youth with these problems are identified during CST evaluations with mental health professionals.[12] Finally, as mentioned by Grisso and colleagues,[11] information about juvenile CST is largely used by the judges who may need guidance making legal decisions regarding young offenders, who may be incompetent to stand trial.

Defendants' CST evaluations often serve as the link between the criminal justice system and biobehavioral sciences, because mental health professionals conduct psychological assessments and provide recommendations to the courts. As already mentioned, competency is a legal issue; however, recommendations provided by various mental health professionals are largely used in the legal decision-making process.[13] As mentioned by Reich and Tookey,[14] recommendations by mental health professionals have an immense influence on judicial determination, with rates of agreement normally exceeding 90%. Accurate assessments of competency are crucial in the legal system, given the large number of unfortunate consequences of erroneous evaluations. For instance, a clinician's failure to identify significant impairments during competency assessments could compromise the fairness of the trial process by limiting the defendant's ability to meaningfully participate in their own defense. Moreover, incorrect identifications of impairment could result in involuntary commitment to a mental health institution and will deprive a defendant of liberty; this can also lead to significant legal problems by substantially slowing the trial process.[15] The role of mental health professionals, specifically psychologists and psychiatrists, is especially important in the area of juvenile adjudicative competence. Most psychological factors, including parental mental health, economic adversity, abuse and neglect, parental criminality, and substance use, are also the same factors responsible for juvenile delinquency and are the same factors implicated in most mental health problems in youths.[16]

The climate surrounding juvenile courts has changed in the last several decades, with an increase in youth being tried in criminal courts and receiving sanctions initially created for adults. These changes were largely instigated by the increases in juvenile crimes in the early 1990s. In response to this dramatic increase in the number of juvenile crimes, more jurisdictions started to move away from the notion of giving shorter and less severe punishments for the youth[3] by making it easier to punish juvenile delinquents.[3,17] Some states, for instance, are making it easier to waive juveniles to an adult court by increasing the range of offenses for which the transfer is allowed and by lowering the age at which juveniles will be allowed to be waived to an adult court.[3] Other changes in the juvenile justice system include mechanisms such as statutory exclusion and prosecutor's direct files, which have become increasingly more prevalent and seek the purpose of providing harsher punishments for juveniles. Given the above-mentioned changes in juvenile justice system regarding juvenile incarcerations, many researchers are starting to raise the question of whether youth in the correctional system have the ability to meaningfully participate in their defense.[5] Consequently, more attention needs to be paid to juveniles in the correctional system and their ability to participate in their own defense. Although the question of juvenile competency is complex, it becomes more difficult when considering the impact of general cognitive development and developmental maturity on competency of youth facing adjudication.

In light of these recent trends in the juvenile justice system, many states are becoming increasingly concerned about young offenders' legal decisional capacity, especially given the high prevalence of psychiatric, developmental, and intellectual disorders in this population. Given the growing number of incarcerated youth with comorbid mental health, and learning and developmental disorders, more research efforts need to be mobilized to understand the impact of comorbidity on juvenile CST status. Although in adult populations CST criteria has mainly concentrated on defendants' mental illnesses or intellectual disabilities, the issue becomes more complex and problematic for the juvenile population where similar problems may manifest due to age, that is, developmental immaturity, rather than mental or psychological illness alone. Therefore, it is essential that mental health professionals working in this area have the appropriate training in child development to complete JCST evaluations. JCST evaluators must pay serious attention to factors, such as age, developmental immaturity, mental illness, and cognitive and learning disorders, because these could serve as risk factors for juvenile incompetency.

CORRELATES OF COMPETENCY TO STAND TRIAL IN JUVENILE OFFENDERS

Competency to Stand Trial and Mental Illness

Youth with psychiatric disorders are overrepresented in delinquent populations, with more than 50% of them displaying some sort of a mental disorder.[7] A study conducted by Baerger and colleagues[5] compared 132 preadjudicated defendants evaluated as IST with 473 petitioned juvenile defendants deemed competent to stand trial. The results showed that most youth deemed IST had been previously determined to have special education needs, had both inpatient and outpatient mental health treatment histories, and had experienced physical/sexual abuse and neglect. Moreover, the study also found that most of the juveniles deemed IST had mental retardation, but in the absence of co-occurring psychiatric disorders. In addition, in a 1995 study, Cowden and Mckee[18] found a correlation between the severity of mental illness diagnosis and the evaluation of competency with youths between 9 and 16 years old. Results indicated that only 28% of youth with severe psychiatric diagnoses were found to be competent, compared with 83% who had a moderate psychiatric diagnosis. In addition, the same study also found that competent and incompetent juveniles could be distinguished on the basis of age, a history of remedial education, and history of mental diagnosis. In 2001, a study of Florida's competency restoration program with juveniles revealed that 58% of those found incompetent to stand trial had a diagnosis of mental retardation; 51% had an Axis I mental health diagnosis of Conduct Disorder, and 57% had psychotic symptoms.[19]

The question of youth competency was further investigated by Christy and colleagues,[20] who conducted a review of 1357 competency evaluations. The review determined that 60% of those declared incompetent were given an Axis I mental diagnosis. To complement these results, preliminary results proposed by Grisso[21] suggested that symptoms of anxiety, depression, and trauma could also significantly diminish the defendant's abilities to participate in the legal process. Symptoms of attention deficit/hyperactivity disorder were also shown to compromise a juvenile's ability to assist the counsel.[22]

Competency to Stand Trial and Age

Historically, age has been one of the major factors influencing juvenile CST status, and therefore, has received considerable research attention. There is a significant body of literature attesting to the fact that juvenile offenders younger than 13 years of age are at an increased risk of being deemed IST, due to their inability to fully comprehend the court procedures. For instance, the first ever published study investigating CST status in the juvenile populations was conducted in 1984 by Savitsky and Karras[10] and investigated the differences between youth and adult population on the scores of Competence Screening Test (for adults) and the Shipley Institute of Living Vocabulary Test. As expected, the researchers found that age was significantly correlated with the scores of above-mentioned measures, such that younger groups were at an increased risk of being deemed incompetent using those measures.[10] In addition, similar results were obtained in another study of 144 juveniles between the ages of 9 and 16 years old. Adolescent age was again significantly correlated with competency, demonstrating that only 18.2% of the 11-year-old participants were considered competent, compared with 72% of those at age 16.

A large-scale study conducted by Grisso and colleagues[11] in 2003 investigated the factors associated with CST status in a group of adolescents between the ages of 11 and 17, and a group of adults ages 18 to 24 across different geographic regions (Los Angeles, northern Florida, southern, northern, and central Virginia). Participants included detained offenders in juvenile facilities and adults jails and community participants who had never been detained before. Consistent with the existing literature in the field, the results indicated that young age was significantly related to reduced competence, showing that participants younger than 13 years old were 3 times more likely to be found incompetent, with one-third of this group failing the competency measures (MacCAT-CA [MacArthur Competence Assessment Tool-Criminal Adjudication] and FIR-R [Fitness Interview Test-Revised]). In comparison, only one-fifth of the 14- to 15-year-old adolescents were deemed incompetent. Furthermore, 16- and 17-year-old participants of the study tested similarly to the adult populations, once again confirming the previous findings, suggesting that young participants are at a significantly increased risk of failing competency measures.[11]

Cognitive Deficits/Learning Disabilities and Competency to Stand Trial

An important predictor of juvenile incompetency is cognitive and intellectual functioning, as a growing body of literature has linked lower levels of cognitive functioning with reduced capacity to participate in court procedures. Research in the area has demonstrated that an Axis II diagnosis of Mental Retardation is highly correlated to IST. A 1980 study by Grisso[23] found that 15 to 19 year olds with an IQ lower than 70 scored poorer on measures of comprehension of defendants' rights compared with 10 to 12 year olds with an average IQ. Similarly, another study found that IQ was significantly related to reduced competency. Forty percent of adolescents who had an IQ between 60 and 74 and 25% of youth who had an IQ between 75 and 89 showed significant impairments in tests measuring competency.[11] The above-mentioned results were further confirmed by other similar studies, which found that youth deemed incompetent to stand trial during CST evaluations had lower intellectual functioning than competent youth,[24,25] displayed higher levels of borderline intellectual functioning and mental retardation[26] and were more likely to be diagnosed with mental retardation than a mental illness.[5]

In addition to low IQ and reduced intellectual functioning, learning disorders and poor academic functioning have also been implicated in reduced competency. The link between cognitive deficits and adjudicative competence has been examined by Warren and colleagues[27] in a sample of 120 psychiatrically hospitalized male adolescents, where learning disorders or mental retardation correlated with low scores of understanding and reasoning on the MacCAT-CA measurement of competency. In addition, according to another study, detained youth who were found IST were more likely to display learning and academic problems than their counterparts who were deemed CST.[5,18,25] These studies provide important preliminary evidence that cognitive development is, in fact, correlated strongly with youth's ability to understand court procedures, make informed decisions, and recognize significant components and factors influencing their case.

MEASUREMENTS

Given the high prevalence of psychiatric conditions in juvenile populations,[7,9] it is not surprising that defense attorneys would have doubts about their clients' abilities to understand the charges against them and meaningfully participate in their own defense. Consequently, competency assessments are one of the most frequently requested forensic assessments in the United States with the estimated 25,000 assessments per year.[28] The consequences of court-ordered forensic evaluations can have significant implications, as incorrect assessments by mental health professionals could compromise the fairness of the trial and lead to unnecessary delays in the criminal justice process. More specifically, incorrect assessments can lead to longer than usual detainment periods, involuntary commitment to public mental health institutions, and consequently, increased financial costs for the public.[15] With these consequences in mind, several measurements have been developed in order to aid mental health professionals in the determining the CST status. Many of these instruments were originally developed for adult populations and are not standardized for youth and adolescent populations. Moreover, these instruments are meant to serve as supplementary tools in the evaluation process, and consequently, cannot be used separately to determine competency status. There are 3 types of assessment instruments in forensic settings: (a) clinical measures and assessment techniques, (b) forensically relevant instruments, and (c) forensic assessment instruments.[6] Clinical measures are psychological test measures developed for assessment, diagnosis, and treatment planning in a therapeutic setting. Forensic relevant instruments address the clinical constructs that are relevant to evaluating individuals within the legal system. Forensic assessment instruments are specifically relevant to legal standards and focus on specific abilities, capacities, and knowledge manifested by law.[6]

MacArthur Competence Assessment Tool-Criminal Adjudication

The MacCAT-CA was developed by the MacArthur Foundation Research network on mental health and the law.[6] It is a highly standardized, 22-item measure that usually takes approximately 45 minutes to complete. The Mac-CAT-CA assesses competency in 3 main subsections: understanding, reasoning, and appreciation. It uses the vignette methodology, which provides an opportunity for the assessors to evaluate the quality of the response through ratings of 2 (adequate), 1 (questionable), or 0 (inadequate).[6] The measure was originally designed for adults, but has been used in studies to compare the competency of juveniles to adult populations.

The Fitness Interview Test-Revised Assesses Understanding, Appreciation, and Communication

FIT-R is a 16-item semistructured clinical interview, which was originally developed for competency assessment in Canadian populations of adult offenders and was based on Canadian standards of CST.[29,30] The interview is flexible and intended to be administered in an ordinary language in order to allow the conversation to flow naturally.[29] Although initially this instrument has not been created to address issues pertaining to developmental maturity and problems created due to adolescent psychosocial development, the simple language used during the assessment makes it suitable for youth assessments as well.[29,30] Consequently, when using FIT-R in juvenile assessment, it is important to keep in mind these limitations and make sure to include questions assessing the above-mentioned domains.

The Juvenile Adjudicative Competence Interview

The Juvenile Adjudicative Competence Interview (JACI) is considered the gold standard for juvenile competency assessments. The primary purpose of the JACI is to ensure that those conducting the examination are collecting relevant information to be considered when the formulating an opinion about a youth's capacity for adjudicative competence.[29] It provides the clinician with a structured set of questions to assess the understanding, appreciation, and reasoning in decisions about rights waiver as it pertains directly to the legal standard for competence to stand trial of the youth.[29,31] The JACI is different from other instruments because it provides the examiner with an opportunity to assess juveniles' immediate as well as long-term retention abilities by first providing them legal related facts and then assessing their knowledge at some later point during the assessment.

The Competence Assessment for Standing Trial for Defendants with Mental Retardation

The CAST-MR (The Competence Assessment for Standing Trial for Defendants with Mental Retardation) is a highly structured clinical interview designed to assess competency of defendants with intellectual disabilities. This instrument was the first instrument designed specifically for those populations, because, despite the extant literature, which documented that intellectual disabilities were related to impairments in competency status, there were no specific assessment instruments that were designed specifically for those populations. The measure contains 50 items divided into 3 sections: basic legal skills, skills to assist the defense, and understanding case events, which separately assess the defendant's knowledge of the legal process, their understanding of the attorney-client relationship, and their ability to communicate the facts of their case.[29,32] Moreover, as mentioned by Kruh and Grisso,[29] although this measure was specifically designed for individuals with intellectual disabilities, the items in the measure are set at a second-grade level, and therefore, could be generalized to the juvenile populations as well.

COMPETENCY RESTORATION

In most states, the question of competence may be raised by the judge, the defense, or the prosecution,[31] and defendants are presumed to be competent unless a doubt is raised. Currently, there is no requirement that all defendants be evaluated and found competent before being allowed to move on with the legal process; however, if, at any point during the legal proceedings concerns arise regarding the defendant's legal capabilities, then the above-mentioned parties have an obligation to raise the question of competency.[33] Moreover, if presented evidence raises a "bona fide doubt," then the judge is obligated to conduct a hearing in the issue, because conviction of the incompetent defendants violates due process.[34] Usually the request for a competency evaluation comes from the judge or the defense attorney,[31] and the court orders a mental health professional to perform an assessment of the defendant's competency status.[33] These evaluations are conducted not only to determine the CST status but also to evaluate the defendant's potential to be restored to competency within a foreseeable period of time with appropriate restoration services.[2,35] These mental health professionals must possess the appropriate knowledge and skill set to conduct the assessments[36] and prepare their findings for the court. Accordingly, most of the time, JCST assessments are conducted by psychologists or psychiatrists with specialized training in forensic assessment and child development and psychopathology.[37]

Typically, when adult defendants are found incompetent to stand trial, they receive treatment and restoration services at a forensic hospital; however, because of the lack of available restoration programs for youth, this process may be more problematic. Once a juvenile is deemed incompetent, the legal proceedings are suspended. In the few jurisdictions where competency restoration programs are available, the judge may require or order restoration services for youth who have been declared incompetent,[16] but these programs are few and far between. Restoration to competency is very challenging in youth and is controversial among experts regarding the best approach. In part, the restoration approach depends on the predicate cause for the finding of incompetency in addition to education on the legal process. In the case of those found incompetent to stand trial due to a mental health disorder, restoration usually involves treating the underlying mental health condition. This treatment process is not different from any other mental health treatment and may require extensive medication treatment along with other psychosocial forms of treatment.[38] For youth who are found IST due to intellectual disability or developmental immaturity, it is more complicated. They may lack the cognitive capacity, development, and maturity to be able to benefit from restoration services. Educational training regarding the legal process is provided, which presents problems for defendants with intellectual disabilities because those people show deficits in their abilities to learn and retain new information.[38] Youth declared incompetent due to mental health problems may receive treatment on either an inpatient or an outpatient basis, whereas those with intellectual and cognitive limitation may be asked to participate in educational training about the legal process, trial details, and various trial outcomes.[16] Furthermore, a judgment needs to be made regarding competency attainment possibilities of youth who were found incompetent based on developmental immaturity alone. In a case where competency attainment is not likely in the foreseeable future, and the offense level is low, the case is dismissed; however, in cases where the minor has committed a violent crime, this poses a challenge for judges, who must balance habeas corpus issues and public safety needs.[16]

Despite the relative paucity of research on restoration programs, recommendations about optimal restoration programs were nevertheless offered by several researchers. For instance, Warren and colleagues,[39] who have one of few published papers on the topic of competency restoration, suggest that the good restoration program must be an individualized, community-based, integrative, and developmentally and culturally appropriate program that is consistent with the current legal standards.[39] Moreover, based on conducted literature review and detailed discussion of clinicians at both the state and the national level, this review[38] presents several key criteria that are necessary for a model competency restoration program. According to the authors, these elements are objective competency assessments before admission, individualized treatment plan with educational and anxiety reduction components, specific educational component for individuals with intellectual limitations, medication treatment, and periodic competency assessments.[38] According to the authors, these elements are only the essential components of a successful restoration program, and therefore, are not meant to be comprehensive. Consequently, it is suggested that each mental health professional dealing with incompetent defendants use these elements and add other available resources to make a successful treatment plan that is unique for the individual.[38]

REFERENCES

1. Dusky v. United States, 362 U.S. 402 (1960).
2. Melton GB, Petrila J, Poythress NG, et al. Psychological evaluations for the courts: a handbook for mental health professionals. New York: Guilford Press; 1997.
3. Grisso T. The competence of adolescents as trial defendants. Psychol Publ Pol Law 1997;3:3–32.
4. In re Gault, 387 U.S. 1 (1967).
5. Baerger DR, Griffin EF, Lyons JS, et al. Competency to stand trial in preadjudicated and petitioned juvenile defendants. J Am Acad Psychiatry Law 2003;31: 314–20.

6. Acklin MW. The forensic clinician's toolbox I: a review of competency to stand trial (CST) instruments. J Pers Assess 2012;94:220–2.
7. Teplin LA, Abram KM, McClelland GM, et al. Psychiatric disorders in youth in juvenile detention. Arch Gen Psychiatry 2002;59:1133–43.
8. Larson KA, Grisso T. National Youth Screening & Assessment Project. Developing Statutes for Competence to Stand Trial in Juvenile Delinquency Proceedings: A Guide for Lawmakers. Center for Mental Health Services Research Publications and Presentations; 2001.
9. Burrel S, Kendrick C, Blalock B. Incompetent youth in California juvenile justice. Stanford Law Pol Rev 2008;19:198–250.
10. Savitsky JC, Karras D. Competency to stand trial among adolescents. Adolescence 1984;19:349–58.
11. Grisso T, Steinberg L, Woolard J, et al. Juveniles' competence to stand trial: a comparison of adolescents' and adults' capacities as trial defendants. Law Hum Behav 2003;27:333–64.
12. Bonnie RJ, Grisso T. Adjudicative competence and youthful offenders. In: Grisso T, Schwartz RG, editors. Youth on trial: a developmental perspective on juvenile justice. Chicago: University of Chicago Press; 2000. p. 73–103.
13. Melton OB, Weithorn LA, Slobogin C. Community mental health centers and the courts: an evaluation of community-based forensic services. Lincoln (NE): University of Nebraska Press; 1985.
14. Reich J, Tookey L. Disagreements between court and psychiatrist on competency to stand trial. J Clin Psychiatry 1986;47:29–30.
15. Hoge SK, Poythress N, Bonnie RJ, et al. The MacArthur adjudicative competence study: diagnosis, psychopathology, and competence-related abilities. Behav Sci Law 1997;15:329–45.
16. Bath E, Gerring J. National trends in juvenile competency to stand trial. J Am Acad Child Adolesc Psychiatry 2014;53:265–8.
17. Geraghty TF, Drizin SA. Foreword-the debate over the future of juvenile courts: can we reach consensus? J Crim Law Criminol 1997;88:1–14.
18. Cowden VL, Mckee GR. Competency to stand trial in juvenile delinquency proceedings – cognitive maturity and the attorney-client relationship. Univ Louisv J Fam Law 1994;33:629–60.
19. McGaha A, Otto RK, McClaren MD, et al. Juveniles adjudicated incompetent to proceed: a descriptive study of Florida's competency restoration program. J Am Acad Psychiatry Law 2001;29:427–37.
20. Christy A, Douglas KS, Otto RK, et al. Juveniles evaluated incompetent to proceed: characteristics and quality of mental health professional's evaluations. Prof Psychol Res Pr 2004;35:380–8.
21. Grisso T. Evaluating juvenile's adjudicative competence: a guide for clinical practice. Sarasota (FL): Professional Resource Press; 2005.
22. Viljoen JL, Roesch R. Competence to waive interrogation rights and adjudicative competence in adolescent defendants: cognitive development, attorney contact, and psychological symptoms. Law Hum Behav 2005;29:723–42.
23. Grisso T. Juveniles' capacities to waive Miranda rights: an empirical analysis. Calif Law Rev 1980;68:1134–66.
24. Evans TM. Juvenile competency to stand trial: problems and pitfalls. Am J Forensic Psychol 2003;21:5–18.
25. Kruh IP, Lynne S, Mesha E, et al. Juvenile competence to stand trial: a historical and empirical analysis of a juvenile forensic evaluation service. Int J Forensic Ment Health 2006;5:109–23.

26. McKee GR, Shea SJ. Competency to stand trial in family court: characteristics of competent and incompetent juveniles. J Am Acad Psychiatry Law 1999;1:65–73.
27. Warren JI, Aaron J, Ryan E, et al. Correlates of adjudicative competence among psychiatrically ill individuals. J Am Acad Psychiatry Law 2003;31:299–309.
28. Steadman HJ, Hartstone E. Defendant's incompetent to stand trial. In: Monahan J, Steadman HJ, editors. Mentally disordered offenders. New York: Plenum; 1983. p. 39–64.
29. Kruh IP, Grisso T. Evaluation of juveniles' competence to stand trial. New York: Oxford University Press; 2008.
30. Roesch R, Zapf PA, Eaves D. Fitness interview test —Revised (FIT-R): a structured, interview for assessing competency to stand trial. Sarasota (FL): Professional Resource Press/Professional Resource Exchange; 2006.
31. Grisso T. Clinical evaluations for juveniles' competence to stand trial: a guide for legal professionals. Sarasota (FL): Professional Resource Press/Professional Resource Exchange; 2005.
32. Everington CT. The competence assessment for standing trial for defendants with mental retardation (Cast-MR) a validation study. Crim Justice Behav 1990;17: 147–68.
33. Grisso T. Evaluating juveniles' adjudicative competence: a guide for clinical practice. Sarasota (FL): Professional Resource Press/Professional Resource Exchange; 2005.
34. Pate v. Robinson, 383 U.S. 375 (1966).
35. Jackson v. Indiana, 406 U.S. 715 (1972).
36. Grisso T. Forensic evaluation of juveniles. Sarasota (FL): Professional Resource Press/Professional Resource Exchange; 1998.
37. Oberlander LB, Goldstein NE, Ho CN. Preadolescent adjudicative competence: methodological considerations and recommendations for practice standards. Behav Sci Law 2001;19:545–63.
38. Noffsinger SG. Restoration to competency practice guidelines. Int J Offender Ther Comp Criminol 2001;45:356–62.
39. Warren JI, DuVal J, Komarovskaya I, et al. Developing a forensic service delivery system for juveniles adjudicated incompetent to stand trial. Int J Forensic Ment Health 2009;8:245–62.

The Role of the Child and Adolescent Psychiatrist in the Adjudicatory Assessment

Camilla L. Lyons, MD, MPH*

KEYWORDS

- Structured professional judgments • Risk assessment • Treatment amenability
- Risk management • Risk communication • Adolescent psychopathy

KEY POINTS

- The use of structured professional judgments is the cornerstone of high-quality forensic evaluations used by the courts to inform legal decisions for adjudicated youth.
- A variety of assessment instruments can be administered by clinician evaluators, including psychiatrists, to optimize the quality of adjudicatory assessments.
- Child and adolescent psychiatrists are in a unique position to apply their diagnostic acumen and expertise in psychopharmacology to adjudicatory assessments.
- Recommended interventions should be evidence-based and readily available in the youth's community; treatment goals should be specific and realistically obtainable.
- If psychopathic traits are identified, the forensic evaluator should consider a description of such traits accompanied by an explicit declaration of the limitations of juvenile psychopathy assessments.

INTRODUCTION

When the courts look to the mental health field to help inform legal decisions, psychiatrists are key members among the skilled mental health clinicians in position to respond. Their expert input is important and offers an opportunity to meaningfully impact the lives of youthful offenders. Means and colleagues[1] found that judges' decisions with regard to transfer of youthful offenders from adult court to juvenile court strongly correlated with the opinion of the forensic evaluator. Campbell and Schmidt[2] found an overall agreement of 67.5% between mental health recommendations and court dispositions.

The author has nothing to disclose.
Department of Psychiatry, New York University School of Medicine, 550 First Avenue, New York, NY 10016, USA
* 26 Village Green, PO Box 296, Bedford, NY 10506.
E-mail address: clyons@aya.yale.edu

Child Adolesc Psychiatric Clin N Am 25 (2016) 61–69
http://dx.doi.org/10.1016/j.chc.2015.08.006 **childpsych.theclinics.com**
1056-4993/16/$ – see front matter

Numerous studies of youth in the juvenile justice system have shown the prevalence of diagnosable mental illness to be 66% to 74%, or two to three times higher than the rate in community samples.[3,4] Given the high burden of illness, youth in the juvenile justice system need high-quality evaluations that are developmentally and psychologically informed. Key components of these evaluations include diagnostic assessment and clarification, risk assessment, estimate of the youth's potential for treatment gains, and specific treatment recommendations.

The American Academy of Child and Adolescent Psychiatry (AACAP) Practice Parameter for Child and Adolescent Forensic Evaluation[5] provides detailed guiding principles that apply to the adjudicatory assessment, among other types of child forensic evaluations. Along with requisite clinic training and skill needed to evaluated clinically complex youth, AACAP advocates that the forensic evaluator also have forensic supervisory training or experience and be knowledgeable about child development and child psychopathology. The evaluator should also be knowledgeable about the relevant, current literature, including the evidence base supporting specific types of treatment and services.

Borum[6] provides further insight on the role of the evaluator in adjudicatory assessments. He explains the need to identify mental health needs in a developmental context and the youth's risk factors for recidivism. Treatment recommendations should identify targets for intervention based on the youth's risk profile. Evaluators' reports must provide the court with a consistent and clear explanation of disposition recommendations. A systematic assessment of risk and needs provides the foundation for effective intervention. The planned interventions should be evidence-based and treatment goals should be realistically obtainable based on the youth's existing capacities. Borum[6] advocates the most intensive monitoring and supervision resources should be reserved for the highest-risk cases. Lastly, the evaluator should provide an implementation plan along with recommendations for frequency of monitoring and reassessment.[6]

KEY COMPONENTS OF ADJUDICATORY ASSESSMENTS

Clinical Needs and Diagnostic Assessment

Clinician reports should include a clinical assessment of the youth, including a Diagnostic and Statistical Manual diagnosis if present, prognosis, and an explanation of how the mental health needs influence the youth's behavior.[7] Much has been written about the mental health screening and assessment of youths in juvenile detention and corrections facilities, including the article by Soulier and McBride.[8] If such tools have been administered to the youth, the results should be reviewed by the clinician evaluator and incorporated into the report. Tests should only be administered, scored, and interpreted by a qualified clinical professional trained in their use, which often includes psychiatrists. Referral for psychological testing should also be considered for diagnostically complex cases or when intellectual disability is suspected.

A commonly used screening tool in this population is the Massachusetts Youth Screening Instrument, Version 2. It is a self-report inventory designed to be administered and scored in about 10 to 15 minutes.[9] In contrast to screening tools, comprehensive assessment instruments usually take longer to administer and are designed to verify the presence or absence of mental health needs among screened-in youths.[9] These tools include the Youth Self-Report, the Diagnostic Interview Schedule for Children-Voice Version (V-DISC), the Minnesota Multiphasic Personality Inventory—Adolescent (MMPI-A), and the Millon Adolescent Clinical Inventory (MACI).[10]

Comprehensive assessment tools provide data needed for diagnostic refinement and specific intervention recommendations.[9] For example, MMPI-A results can help evaluate an adolescent's current willingness to engage in treatment, need for structure, and capacity for impulse control; the MMPI-A results should be viewed as a cross-sectional assessment of a youth's psychological functioning at the time the tool was administered.[11] The MACI assists in the assessment of general psychopathology, peer difficulties, confusion about self, family problems, and a youth's strengths and weaknesses. The MACI also assists in identifying youth that are more likely to exhibit oppositional behaviors and suicidal behaviors.[12]

Risk Assessment for Future Offending

Assessments of adjudicated youth should include a systematic and developmentally informed review of the youth's risk factors for recidivism. There are three approaches to assessing risk of violence: (1) unstructured clinical judgment, (2) actuarial judgment, and (3) structured professional judgment. The latter is preferable in that it addresses the limitations of the other two approaches and emphasizes prevention over prediction of future offending.[13] There is growing support for less reliance on intuition when assessing risk and needs of youth in the juvenile justice system and more use of structured decision-making instruments.[14–16] Research shows that risk ratings based on structured clinical assessments perform better than unstructured clinical judgments and may perform better than some actuarial predictions.[17]

The use of a structured professional judgment instrument, such as the Structured Assessment of Violence Risk in Youth (SAVRY) and Youth Level of Service/Case Management Inventory (YLS/CMI), ensures that the evaluator's needs assessment and management recommendations are anchored by a systematic review of static and dynamic risk factors and then filtered through a lens of clinical wisdom.[14]

The SAVRY is an instrument designed to structure and improve the practice of risk assessment and risk management among youth in juvenile justice settings, while drawing on the existing research base. By design, it is systematic, empirically grounded, developmentally informed, treatment oriented, flexible, and practical. In general, psychologists, psychiatrists, trained juvenile probation officers, and social workers with requisite expertise (including child and adolescent development and youth violence) are qualified to the use the SAVRY, which does not require a training course. The SAVRY protocol is composed of six items defining protective factors and 24 items defining risk factors, which are further broken down into three subcategories (historical, individual, and social/contextual). For each risk factor item the manual contains specific guidelines for rating the severity according to a three-level nonnumeric coding structure (high, moderate, and low). Protective factors are coded as present or absent. The evaluator must weigh the relevance of each factor to the particular youth and reach an opinion about the nature and degree of the youth's violence risk.[18]

The YLS/CMI is a standardized inventory for use with juvenile offenders. It assesses factors associated with risk of recidivism and need factors that assist in case management. A probation officer or other trained professional can complete the YLS/CMI. The YLS/CMI is based on three principles of case classification. The risk principle states that the intensity of services should be matched to the level of risk. The need principle states that targets of service should reflect the criminogenic needs, or dynamic risk factors, of the youth. The responsivity principle states that decisions about interventions should incorporate factors that may not directly impact criminal activity but remain relevant, such as intellectual disability, motivation for treatment, emotional maturity, prosocial attitudes, and support from adults.[19]

Amenability to Treatment

As *Kent v United States*[20] lays out, the "sophistication and maturity" and the "likelihood of reasonable rehabilitation of the juvenile" should be factored into the decision about the transfer of juvenile cases to adult court. Salekin and colleagues[21] propose that constructs delineated in *Kent* can be applied to a broader range of dispositional cases. Again, there is a role for a structured professional judgment approach in assessing treatment amenability. The Risk-Sophistication-Treatment Inventory (RSTI) was designed to meet the specific needs of mental health professionals who provide dispositional and transfer assessments for the juvenile courts. The RSTI can be used before disposition decisions or to assist with legal decisions about treatment and design of individualized treatment plans.[21] It is composed of three scales: (1) risk for dangerousness, (2) sophistication-maturity, and (3) treatment amenability. Child and adolescent psychiatrists who receive training on the instrument to ensure rating reliability are eligible to administer the RSTI (Randall Salekin, personal communication, 2015).

The risk for dangerousness scale items focus on characteristics that reflect a violent history, frequent involvement in criminal activity, premeditation, leadership role in crimes, and lack of remorse and general disregard for others. The sophistication-maturity scale items reflect levels of autonomy, internal locus of control, decision-making capacities, and degree of emotional attunement. This includes an assessment of awareness of the wrongfulness of crimes, ability to generate and weigh alternatives, future time perspective or foresight, ability to delay gratification, emotional self-regulation skills, conflict resolution skills, and self-reflection skills. The treatment amenability scale items reflect the degree and type of psychopathology, motivation to engage in treatment, expectations that treatment will be beneficial, anxiety about one's current situation, positive involvement by parents, awareness of one's problems, a sense of responsibility for one's actions, guilt or remorse, openness to change, and positive attachments.[22]

Risk Management and Treatment Recommendations

Evaluators should highlight for the court specific treatment targets and prioritize them based on the extent to which they may reduce risk for recidivism.[6] Dowden and Andrews[23] found that programs that focused primarily on criminogenic factors showed larger effect sizes in reducing reoffending. These factors included family supervision, self-control, anger, and academics.[6,23]

Once treatment targets are identified, the evaluator should specify the modality, frequency, and setting of treatment being recommended. This requires that the evaluator have a strong working knowledge of the resources in the youth's community.[7] Wherever possible, evaluators should recommend treatment programs that are evidenced-based, including multisystemic therapy, functional family therapy, and multidimensional treatment foster care.[6,24] Specifically, cognitive behavioral treatments should be considered because they show stronger effects in reducing recidivism than pure behavior modification strategies.[6,25] Intensive interventions should be reserved for the highest-risk cases.[6] Again, these resources must be accessible to the youth in question; although it may be academically satisfying to recommend to the court a full menu of wraparound services for a particular youth, it is not necessarily helpful to the court if such modalities are not available to the youth because of geography, insurance coverage, waiting lists, or other barriers.

Additionally, the length of a youth's placement and/or probation term limits the window for supervised treatment. This may be a relatively short period of time and evaluators must remain mindful about what treatment goals can realistically be accomplished during the given time frame.

Child and adolescent psychiatrists are in a unique position to provide psychopharmacologic treatment recommendations when indicated. This population has high rates of diagnosable mental illness. Still, youth in juvenile justice facilities may not be receiving psychopharmacologic interventions at rates commensurate with prevalence of mental illness. Lyons and colleagues[26] reported that in a sample of youth in secure detention, only 21% of those who endorsed an anxiety disorder, a mood disorder, or attention deficit/hyperactivity disorder on V-DISC were prescribed a psychotropic medication during their first month of stay. Youths at risk for persistent serious delinquency are less likely to have received treatment in their communities,[27] and their entry into the juvenile justice system represents an opportunity for access to mental health care.[28–30] Psychiatrist evaluators should seize this opportunity to recommend the start of much-needed treatment when indicated.

The evaluator may consider recommending when reassessments of risk and need should be conducted. Adolescents are moving targets in terms of cognition, biology, and social-emotional functioning. They must be reassessed to ensure that treatment plans are modified in response to changing needs and risk factors.[6] If monitoring is being recommended, the evaluator should specify where and how that monitoring should take place,[6] including who should collect the data and which data are needed.

CLINICAL PEARLS AND PRACTICE GUIDELINES

Scope of Assessment and Evaluator's Role

The forensic evaluator should only answer the question being asked. Furthermore, the evaluator's opinion should not go beyond the scope of one's professional training. The evaluator's task is to provide information and opinions that may inform legal decisions but not to provide an opinion on the ultimate legal issue.[17]

Sometimes the clinician providing treatment to a youth within the juvenile justice system is asked to step into the role of forensic evaluator. This dual role should be avoided whenever possible because it may undermine treatment alliance and therapeutic neutrality.[31] AACAP Practice Parameter[5] provides additional guidance to the treating clinician who is called on by the court to serve as a fact witness, rather than as an expert witness.

Communication of Risk

As Borum and Verhaagen[17] point out, the shift from violence prediction to risk assessment did not occur until the 1980s and it was not until the 1990s that the topic of risk communication was systematically examined. Borum and Verhaagen[17] describe three of the most common forms of risk communication: (1) descriptive, (2) prediction-oriented, and (3) management-oriented. The descriptive style lists the risk factors and does not draw any conclusions about the likelihood of future offending. The predictive style makes a direct statement about the degree of risk of likelihood of future offending; Borum and Verhaagen[17] suggest the use of relative risk in comparison with a particular group within a given time-frame. The management-oriented style or risk reduction approach is the one most highly valued by clinicians, especially in high-risk cases. The management-oriented approach includes an assessment of a specific type of violence that a youth might commit contingent on a set of risk factors, and then describes how those factors may be modified or mitigated with specific interventions.[17]

Psychopathy

There is considerable debate about labeling psychopathic traits in adolescents, particularly those involved in the juvenile justice system.[32] On the one hand, identifying youth with psychopathic traits predicts recidivism. Multiple studies have found that psychopathic traits, identified using the Psychopathy Checklist: Youth Version, predicted violent recidivism.[33–35] Furthermore, longitudinal research shows that a small proportion of early male delinquents go on to commit more than 50% of all crime.[36] The prospect of identifying those youth early on represents substantial potential benefit in terms of public safety. On the other hand, the psychopathy label may be prejudicial and psychopathic traits may not be stable over time. Jones and Cauffman[37] found that psychopathic traits in juveniles had a pejorative influence on legal proceedings, leading to higher perception of dangerousness among judges and more restrictive placements. Furthermore, some adolescents who display psychopathic traits do not go on to become adult psychopaths.[17]

Still, there may be a middle ground. Identification of psychopathic traits in juveniles may also represent an opportunity to identify developmental antecedents of the psychopathy construct and to intervene at a time when traits may be more mutable.[38] Although Salekin cautions against labeling a youth as "psychopathic," he also argues that adolescent offenders with psychopathic traits should not be dismissed as untreatable.[39,40] Treatment of youth with psychopathic traits has been shown to have a positive effect.[39,41–43] If psychopathic traits are identified, the forensic evaluator should consider a description of such traits accompanied by an explicit clarification of the limitations of extending the construct of psychopathy downward to juveniles and limitations of psychopathy assessments.[40] A survey of forensic clinicians found that most describe the characteristics associated with psychopathy if they are present, whether or not they explicitly refer to them as psychopathy related.[44] The evaluator must convey that the presence of psychopathic traits in youth is neither a prediction of adult psychopathy, nor a harbinger of treatment failure. To the contrary, there is concern about the longer-term stability of these traits,[45] and there is evidence to support the positive effect of treatment on recidivism.[39]

SUMMARY

Youths in the juvenile justice system have a high burden of mental illness and courts look to mental health clinicians for guidance to inform legal decisions. Evaluating youth for adjudicatory assessments represents a distinct opportunity for psychiatrists, among other high-skilled clinicians, to comprehensively assess these justice-involved youth for psychiatric diagnosis, risk of recidivism, treatment needs, and treatment amenability. Adjudicated youth are likely to benefit when evaluators use structured professional judgment tools to inform their assessments and recommendations. There is potential for clinician evaluators to play a key role in the reduction of crime, thereby benefiting not only the lives of individual youths but also the greater public.

ACKNOWLEDGMENTS

The author acknowledges insightful discussions with the Honorable Monica Drinane, the Honorable Daniel Turbow, and Dr Adria Adams, PsyD.

REFERENCES

1. Means RF, Heller LD, Janofsky JS. Transferring juvenile defendants from adult to juvenile court: how Maryland forensic evaluators and judges reach their decisions. J Am Acad Psychiatry Law 2012;40(3):333–40.
2. Campbell MA, Schmidt F. Comparison of mental health and legal factors in the disposition outcome of young offenders. Crim Justice Behav 2000;27(6):688–715.
3. Teplin L, Abram K, McClelland G, et al. Psychiatric disorders in youth in juvenile detention. Arch Gen Psychiatry 2002;59(12):1133–43.
4. Wasserman GA, McReynolds LS, Lucas CP, et al. The voice DISC-IV with incarcerated male youths: prevalence of disorder. J Am Acad Child Adolesc Psychiatry 2002;41(3):314–21.
5. Kraus LJ, Thomas CR, Bukstein OG, et al. Practice parameter for child and adolescent forensic evaluation. J Am Acad Child Adolesc Psychiatry 2011;50(12):1299–312.
6. Borum R. Managing at-risk juvenile offenders in the community: putting evidenced based principles into practice. Mental Health Law & Policy Faculty Publications; 2003. p. 47. Available at: http://scholarcommons.usf.edu/mhlp_facpub/47.
7. Kraus LJ, Sobel H. Post-adjudicatory assessment of youth. In: Kessler CL, Kraus LJ, editors. The mental health needs of young offenders: forging paths toward reintegration and rehabilitation. New York: Cambridge University Press; 2007. p. 423–36.
8. Soulier M, McBride A. Mental health screening and assessment of detained youth. Child Adolesc Psychiatric Clin N Am 2015, in press.
9. Grisso T. Why we need mental health screening and assessment in juvenile justice programs. In: Grisso T, Vincent G, Seagrave D, editors. Mental health screening and assessment in juvenile justice. New York: The Guilford Press; 2005. p. 3–21.
10. Grisso T. Comprehensive assessment instruments. In: Grisso T, Vincent GM, Seagrave D, editors. Mental health screening and assessment in juvenile justice. New York: The Guilford Press; 2005. p. 185–6.
11. Archer RP, Baker EM. Minnesota multiphasic personality inventory–adolescent. In: Grisso T, Vincent GM, Seagrave D, editors. Mental health screening and assessment in juvenile justice. New York: The Guilford Press; 2005. p. 240–52.
12. Salekin RT, Leistico AM, Schrum CL, et al. Millon adolescent clinical inventory. In: Grisso T, Vincent GM, Seagrave D, editors. Mental health screening and assessment in juvenile justice. New York: The Guilford Press; 2005. p. 253–64.
13. Grisso T. Risk for violence and recidivism assessment tools. In: Grisso T, Vincent GM, Seagrave D, editors. Mental health screening and assessment in juvenile justice. New York: The Guilford Press; 2005. p. 265–9.
14. Mulvey EP, Iselin AM. Improving professional judgments of risk and amenability in juvenile justice. Future Child 2008;18(2):35–57.
15. Borum R. Assessing violence risk among youth. J Clin Psychol 2000;56(10):1263–88.
16. Hoge RD. Standardized instruments for assessing risk and need in youthful offenders. Crim Justice Behav 2002;29(4):380–96.
17. Borum R, Verhaagen D. Assessing and managing violence risk in juveniles. New York: The Guildford Press; 2006.
18. Borum R, Bartel PA, Forth AE. Structured assessment of violence risk in youth. In: Grisso T, Vincent GM, Seagrave D, editors. Mental health screening and assessment in juvenile justice. New York: The Guilford Press; 2005. p. 311–23.

19. Hoge RD. Youth level of service/case management inventory. In: Grisso T, Vincent GM, Seagrave D, editors. Mental health screening and assessment in juvenile justice. New York: The Guilford Press; 2005. p. 283–94.
20. *Kent v United States*, 383 U.S. 541 (1966).
21. Salekin RT, Salekin KL, Clements CB, et al. Risk-sophistication-treatment inventory. In: Grisso T, Vincent GM, Seagrave D, editors. Mental health screening and assessment in juvenile justice. New York: The Guilford Press; 2005. p. 341–56.
22. Salekin RT. Risk-sophistication-treatment inventory professional manual. Lutz (FL): Psychological Assessment Resources, Inc; 2004.
23. Dowden C, Andrews DA. What works in young offender treatment: a meta-analysis. Forum on Corrections Research 1999;11(2):21–4.
24. Henggeler SW, Sheidow AJ. Empirically supported family-based treatments for conduct disorder and delinquency in adolescents. J Marital Fam Ther 2012; 38(1):30–58.
25. Pearson FS, Lipton DS, Cleland CM, et al. The effects of behavioral/cognitive-behavioral programs on recidivism. Crime Delinquen 2002;48(3):476–96.
26. Lyons CL, Wasserman GA, Olfson M, et al. Psychotropic medication patterns among youth in juvenile justice. Adm Policy Ment Health 2013;40(2):58–68.
27. Hazen AL, Hough RL, Landsverk JA, et al. Use of mental health services by youths in public sectors of care. Ment Health Serv Res 2004;6(4):213–26.
28. Desai RA, Goulet JL, Robbins J, et al. Mental health care in juvenile detention facilities: a review. J Am Acad Psychiatry Law 2006;34(2):204–14.
29. Farmer EM, Burns BJ, Phillips SD, et al. Pathways into and through mental health services for children and adolescents. Psychiatr Serv 2003;54(1):60–6.
30. Chapman JF, Desai RA, Falzer PR. Mental health service provision in juvenile justice facilities: pre- and postrelease psychiatric care. Child Adolesc Psychiatr Clin N Am 2006;15(2):445–58.
31. Strasburger LH, Gutheil TG, Brodsky A. On wearing two hats: role conflict in serving as both psychotherapist and expert witness. Am J Psychiatry 1997; 154(4):448–56.
32. Petrila J, Skeem JL. An introduction to the special issues on juvenile psychopathy and some reflections on the current debate. Juvenile psychopathy: the debate. Behav Sci Law 2003;21(6):689–94.
33. Corrado RR, Vincent GM, Hart SD, et al. Predictive validity of the psychopathy checklist: youth version for general and violent recidivism. Behav Sci Law 2004;22(1):5–22.
34. Gretton HM, Hare RD, Catchpole RE. Psychopathy and offending from adolescent to adulthood: a 10-year follow-up. J Consult Clin Psychol 2004;72(4):636–45.
35. Salekin RT, Leistico AM, Neumann CS, et al. Psychopathy and comorbidity in a young offender sample: taking a closer look at psychopathy's potential importance over disruptive behavior disorders. J Abnorm Psychol 2004;113(3):416–27.
36. Moffitt TE. Adolescence-limited and life-course-persistent antisocial behavior: a developmental taxonomy. Psychol Rev 1993;100(4):674–701.
37. Jones S, Cauffman E. Juvenile psychopathy and judicial decisions making: an empirical analysis of an ethical dilemma. Behav Sci Law 2008;26(2):151–65.
38. DaSilva DR, Rijo D, Salekin RT. Child and adolescent psychopathy: a state-of-the-art reflection on the construct and etiological theories. J Crim Justice 2012;40(4): 269–77.
39. Salekin RT. Psychopathy and therapeutic pessimism: clinical lore or clinical reality? Clin Psychol Rev 2002;22(1):79–112.

40. Vitacco MJ, Salekin RT. Adolescent psychopathy and the law. In: Kiehl KA, Sinnott-Armstrong W, editors. Handbook on psychopathy and the law. New York: Oxford University Press; 2013. p. 78–89.
41. Salekin RT, Worley CB, Grimes RD. Treatment of psychopathy: a review and brief introduction to the mental models approach. Behav Sci Law 2010;28(2):235–66.
42. Caldwell MF, Skeem JL, Salekin RT, et al. Treatment response of adolescent offenders with psychopathy features: a 2-year follow-up. Crim Justice Behav 2006;33(5):571–96.
43. Caldwell MF, McCormick DJ, Umstead D, et al. Evidence of treatment progress and therapeutic outcomes among adolescents with psychopathic features. Crim Justice Behav 2007;34(5):573–87.
44. Viljoen JL, McLachlan K, Vincent GM. Assessing violence risk and psychopathy in juvenile and adult offenders: a survey of clinical practices. Assessment 2010; 17(3):377–95.
45. Salekin RT, Frick PJ. Psychopathy in children and adolescents: the need for a developmental perspective. J Abnorm Child Psychol 2005;33(4):403–9.

Mental Health Care of Detained Youth and Solitary Confinement and Restraint Within Juvenile Detention Facilities

Kevin Whitley, MD, MA[a], John S. Rozel, MD, MSL[b,c,*]

KEYWORDS

• Mental health treatment • Juvenile justice • Juvenile detention
• Trauma-informed care • Solitary confinement • Isolation • Seclusion

KEY POINTS

- Youth in the juvenile justice system have a high prevalence of a diverse array of mental disorders and severe psychosocial stressors.
- Trauma is common and trauma-informed care should be considered a universal precaution in working with justice-involved youth.
- Youth can benefit significantly from evidence-based psychosocial and pharmacologic interventions.
- Although clinically ordered and supervised seclusion may be appropriate in limited situations, disciplinary or punitive use of isolation or solitary confinement is categorically inappropriate.

INTRODUCTION

Mental health treatment of juvenile offenders provides a unique opportunity for treatment providers. Although the work may be challenging, the clinical needs and opportunities for early and meaningful interventions are significant. Adjudication "is the court process that determines (judges) if the juvenile committed the act for which he or she is charged. The term 'adjudicated' is analogous to 'convicted' and indicates that the

---

Disclosure: The authors have nothing to disclose.
[a] Southwood Psychiatric Hospital, 2575 Boyce Plaza Road, Pittsburgh, PA 15241, USA; [b] Shuman Detention Center, Pittsburgh, PA, USA; [c] Re:solve Crisis Network, 333 North Braddock Avenue, Pittsburgh, PA 15208, USA
* Corresponding author. Re:solve Crisis Network, 333 North Braddock Avenue, Pittsburgh, PA 15208.
E-mail address: rozeljs@upmc.edu

Child Adolesc Psychiatric Clin N Am 25 (2016) 71–80
http://dx.doi.org/10.1016/j.chc.2015.08.003
childpsych.theclinics.com
1056-4993/16/$ – see front matter

court concluded the juvenile committed the act."[1] Youth are most often adjudicated for violence directed at others, vandalism, burglary or robbery, status offenses including curfew violation, loitering or disorderly conduct, truancy, running away, underage drinking, trespassing, weapons offenses, drug abuse violations, and driving under the influence. Less common reasons for adjudication include aggravated assault, homicide, manslaughter, arson, gambling, embezzlement, forgery, counterfeiting, prostitution, obstruction of justice, and sexual deviance.

Many reasons for the adjudication of youth exist. Often the youths' causes for adjudication are complex: comorbid psychosocial conditions and stressors are common. Youthful offenses are frequently influenced by poverty, disenfranchisement, poor access to jobs, residential segregation, schools ill-equipped to address acting-out behaviors, family structure including single-parent households and family disruption or a parent in prison, substance use, mental health disorders, and so forth. Community-level structural factors impede systemic social organizations and often impede living within the constraints of the law.

Mental health care of youth involved in the juvenile justice system provides a unique opportunity to approach and remedy social constraints and psychiatric illness. Adjudicated youth have significantly higher rates of mental illness than youth in the general population. The prevalence of mental health disorders in adjudicated youth in nonresidential facilities is estimated to be 50%.[2] The prevalence of mental illness among youth involved in the juvenile justice system located in residential treatment facilities is estimated to be between 65% and 70%.[3] Youth in the juvenile justice system can have any illness within the spectrum of mental illness. Behavioral disorders like conduct disorder are the most frequently diagnosed mental illnesses in adjudicated youth at 46.5%[3] and 62% for male youth and 48% of female youth.[4] Substance use disorders occur in 46.2% of adjudicated youth.[3] Anxiety disorders are estimated to affect 34.4% of youth in the juvenile justice system,[3] and 18.3% of adjudicated youth have mood disorders (according to Wasserman and colleagues[3]). Fazel and colleagues[4] reported that 10.6% of male youth and 29.2% of female youth have clinical depression. Attention-deficit/hyperactivity disorder prevalence is measured at 21% for male youth and 24% for female youth. In addition, it is estimated that up to 19% of detained youths are suicidal, and approximately 50% of female youth in juvenile justice system have symptoms of posttraumatic stress disorder (PTSD). It is common for youth to have more than one mental disorder. When conduct disorder is removed as a possible mental disorder in adjudicated youth, 66.3% of youth meet criteria for a mental disorder.[5]

The problems adjudicated children face are diverse. Each child's social and mental health needs are unique. Despite the heterogeneity of the problems faced by adjudicated youth, mental health treatment has been shown to reduce recidivism rates by 25% compared with children who are not treated for psychiatric illness.[6] The most successful programs have reduced recidivism rates by 25% to 80%.[7]

PRINCIPLES OF ADJUDICATED YOUTH MENTAL HEALTH TREATMENT

Juvenile court provides access to mental and physical health treatment, social services, family-based services, and educational services. The services provided should be child and family focused, culturally competent, and community based. Treatment should coordinate and collaborate with all integrated systems of care to create a unique and individualized treatment approach. However, resources provided to adjudicated youth often try to fix the youth and the individual problems faced without taking into account the family's needs, the community, and the culture. Furthermore, families are often blamed for needing social and mental health services. Attitudes of treatment providers, the court, and society at large blame families for their difficulties. Problem-based treatment by providers, a family's inability to access beneficial services, lack of service responsiveness, and blame often cause families to become frustrated and upset, leaving them less able to address family difficulties and more vulnerable to hardship.

The National Mental Health Association identified a series of values and principles inherent to the care of children in the juvenile justice system in the publication *Mental Health Treatment for Youth in the Juvenile Justice System: A Compendium of Promising Practices* (2004):

- Early identification and intervention are vital to promoting positive outcomes.
- Children must have access to a comprehensive array of individualized formal and informal services that address their physical, emotional, social, and educational needs.
- Services should be delivered in the least restrictive, normative environment that is clinically appropriate.
- Families and care givers should be full participants in all aspects of policy development and the planning and delivery of services, which should be integrated with linkages between child and family serving agencies and programs.
- Care coordination should be provided to ensure that multiple services are linked and clinically indicated. They should also address a family's strengths and needs, and be reviewed on a regular basis for applicability to the family's current level of functioning.
- The service delivery system should include providers who help enable smooth transitions to adult services, if necessary.
- The rights of children should be protected and effective advocacy efforts should be promoted.
- Services must be provided without regard to race, religion, national origin, sex, physical disability, or similar characteristics.

This system is a public health–based model of care that attempts to move away from punitive measures. This system of care offers comprehensive, flexible, and tailored treatment and support to youths and families in the juvenile detention system. The needs of these youth and families are complex. No specific organization can adequately address all the treatment needs that families face. When the treatment needs of families are adequately met, youth spend less time in the legal system and more time with their families, which helps to support the development of healthy and productive families.

TRAUMA ISSUES IN JUVENILE JUSTICE

Numerous studies have identified high rates of PTSD, trauma, and polytrauma in adjudicated youth.[8,9] Sexual trauma in particular is seen as a major risk factor for justice involvement for young female youth in general and female youth of color in particular.[10] Although clinicians working with youth in any acute psychiatric setting are likely already familiar with trauma-informed work, there are additional factors making trauma-informed care for adjudicated youth more challenging, which are addressed here.

One of the most significant limitations of trauma work in juvenile justice settings is the stability of the therapeutic relationship. Trauma-focused treatment is generally recognized to be most effective when it occurs in a stable, safe therapeutic setting in which the youth feels comfortable beginning to discuss the traumatic experiences.[11,12] These factors are often hampered by the juvenile justice system in several ways, including lack of clinical control over length of treatment, lack of clinical control over the environment of care or custody, and potential conflicts of interest that may arise when details of traumatic experiences reveal details about criminal conduct of the youth or others that may be reportable or the subject of an ongoing criminal case. Traumatic exposures may also include experiences in placement or foster care, including physical or sexual assault or witnessing the assault of other youth.

Traumatic experiences of youth in juvenile justice systems may differ qualitatively and quantitatively from the experiences of other youth. In the authors' direct clinical experience at a juvenile detention center, violent bereavement and violent victimization are frequent causes of trauma. The traumatic losses may be the result of sudden death of family members or peers from severe illness or acquired immunodeficiency syndrome, drug use, or violent crime. Repeated traumatization is common and one study identified that 5% of incarcerated youth have had 11 or more major traumatic experiences.[9]

In addition, trauma-related symptoms can be misinterpreted as disciplinary issues by criminal justice professionals; for example, exaggerated startle responses misperceived as aggression, and dissociative freezing misperceived as noncompliance. When severe, chronic, or linked to early childhood traumas, PTSD can mimic many other psychiatric disorders. Complex, chronic, and early childhood traumas can also have profound impacts on subsequent neurodevelopment and functioning.[13,14] Although there are many trauma-focused juvenile justice placements that excel in managing youth with trauma and PTSD issues, many other settings still face or even create many challenges in working with traumatized youth.

Effective treatment of trauma involves medications and psychotherapy and should occur in the context of a therapeutic relationship that is stable and experienced as safe for the consumer. That context is not possible in many juvenile justice settings. Although some residential treatment programs may be able to provide trauma-informed if not trauma-focused interventions, many settings are unable to meet those standards. In ersatz settings, consider the axiom that a clinician should screen for symptoms, not dive for details. That is, a good interview detailing the severity and frequency of PTSD symptoms can be obtained without delving into the especially painful details of the trauma. At the least, giving the youth permission to end the line of questioning at any time is encouraged. In addition, clinicians should consider trauma-informed care as a universal precaution: trauma is so prevalent in this population that it is prudent to assume that any youth may have an undisclosed trauma history.[15]

CRISIS MANAGEMENT OF YOUTH IN DETENTION CENTERS

Many adjudicated youth are detained in detention centers. Detained youth are often new to the detention process, scared, and carry a diagnosis of psychiatric illness. The risk for suicide and self-injurious behavior among these youth is high. Current suicidal thoughts, recent suicidal behavior, and current passive death wish or hopelessness are common in incarcerated youth and are spontaneously reported only half of the time.[16] A primary goal of all detention centers is to maintain the safety and welfare of all youth within the facility. Detention facilities should act quickly and efficiently when a mental health crisis arises by protecting youth from self-injurious behavior and suicide.

New residents should be screened for suicidality, self-injurious thoughts, and past and current psychiatric treatment by trained staff familiar with mental health procedures and needs. Self-injurious behavior is minimized when mental health assessments occur before presentation to the treatment facility by a crisis management team or immediately after presentation to the detention center. In addition, completion of a written screening assessment, like the MAYSI (Massachusetts Youth Screening Instrument), within 48 hours helps to identify youth at risks for self-harm. Prompt referral to mental health clinicians minimizes the chance of harm when the screening assessment indicates a risk for suicide. All detention center staff are trained on how to identify youth at risk of self-harm and expected to observe all youth for self-injurious behavior and risk for suicide. If safety concerns for a resident arise an urgent assessment is completed by a mental health clinician.

When a resident is identified as a suicide risk supportive supervision of the resident is mandated. Supervision is best organized and understood by detention facility staff when the same procedures apply to all residents identified in need of supervision. Supervision is a tiered process that slowly reinstates independence while providing emotional support. One-on-one observation is the most restrictive precaution, and is reserved for individuals who are imminently suicidal or homicidal. Residents on one-to-one observation present a risk for harm. The staff member must remain within a predefined distance from the resident to best protect the resident from harm. Usually, this distance is defined as within 1 m (3 feet) or arm's length. Residents on one-to-one observation may be required to remain in their rooms. When allowed out of their rooms, additional vigilance is needed to assure that the residents cannot evade observing staff member and injure themselves. The residents should be educated on detention facility policies with regard to observation and provided with supportive listening by the staff observer and a mental health clinician. The residents work with the mental health clinicians to determine the best time to discontinue one-on-one observation with close supervision. When a resident feels safe, the resident is allowed more freedom, with a goal of safely mainstreaming the resident into activities. The resident continues to be watched constantly from a distance. If the mental health team is concerned a resident may become, or is, suicidal without the resident admitting to self-injurious thoughts, detention facility staff document the safety of the resident hourly. If further concerns for the safety of the resident arise, prompt actions to protect the resident from harm can be obtained. All residents identified with the potential for self-harm are discussed by the mental health treatment team on a daily basis. Safety issues and elimination of restrictions are addressed promptly. Although care must be taken to minimize the impact of youth malingering suicidality to avoid detention, it is also reasonable to consider emergency psychiatric evaluation or admission in some situations.

DISORDERS COMMONLY ASSOCIATED WITH DELINQUENT YOUTH

Some specific disorders are of particular concern in juvenile justice settings. Almost by definition, most youth entering the juvenile justice system have some pattern of behavior that threatens the physical, financial, or emotional welfare of others. It is common for youth to enter the legal system after committing acts of battery, assault, vandalism, or other acts that jeopardize the rights of others. If there is a pattern of aggressive, deceitful, dangerous, or difficult behavior that violates social norms and creates conflict with individuals in a position of authority, a diagnosis of disruptive, impulse control, and conduct disorder should be considered.[17(p461)]

Up to 75% of children in the legal system have social skills deficits.[18] Treating disruptive, impulse control, and conduct disorders often proves challenging. Research shows that children with significant disruptive behavior benefit from skills-based interventions,[19] parenting/teacher skills training, group therapy, and behavioral therapy to improve peer interactions and compliance with requests from authority figures.[20] Behavioral therapy should focus on problem-solving skills and social competence.[21]

Because of parent detachment in the adjudicated youth population, family involvement in treatment is not always an option.

Social skills training often includes these core functions:

- Social skills acquisition
- Vocational training
- Academic assistance and direction
- Life skills acquisition

Any youth who is noncompliant with treatment and repeatedly places others at risk of harm, even if the risk of harm is mild, should be considered for treatment in a residential treatment facility. Adequate residential facility treatment entails a multiple-phase program. Successful residential treatment programs are often cognitive behavior therapy focused and include, but are not limited to: (1) social skill training, (2) anger management, and (3) moral reasoning. Each phase is multipronged. The programs average around 10 weeks in duration, but can take up to 2 years to complete, especially if the child has a severe pattern of conduct disorder behavior or low intelligence quotient.

A core treatment model for a residential program for adjudicated youth may include:

Social skills training[22]

- Take responsibility for actions: accept that actions have consequences, acknowledge and express feelings, eliminate negative thoughts, focus on positive thoughts, act responsibly, adequate hygiene
- Environmental behaviors: understand how the environment affects behaviors, how to act in an emergency, target problematic areas like the lunchroom
- Task-related behaviors: ask questions, follow direction, acknowledge consequences to actions before acting, complete tasks, participate in groups, work independently, work quality
- Interpersonal behaviors: accepting authority, understanding conflict and consequences, greeting and helping others, talking to others, appropriate play, maintaining a positive attitude

Anger management

- Define anger: what triggers or causes anger, actions associated with anger, factors that complicate anger
- Control of anger: early signs of anger, how to control anger, how not to act
- Strategies to control anger: assertive actions, appropriate self-care, strategies to overcome anger, responding in a nonviolent manner
- Relationships: controlling anger in relationships, improve communication
- Understanding thought distortion: recognize and challenge negative thoughts, focus on healthy thoughts, consider situations that result in anger
- Challenges to controlling anger: difficulties when changing behavior, how to address setbacks

Moral reasoning

- Logic building: determine what is fair and just, and right and wrong
- Empathy building: acknowledge rights of others and what it is like to walk in their shoes
- Learn how to help others

In addition to behavioral therapy, family therapy, and treatment in a residential treatment facility, there is evidence that medications improve symptoms of disruptive, impulse control, and conduct disorders. At present there are no US Food and Drug Administration–approved medications to help guide treatment in this population.

MEDICATION MANAGEMENT

A large percentage of adjudicated youth are diagnosed with mental illnesses besides disruptive behavior disorders. Psychiatric medication management is common within this population. Despite the frequency of treatment with psychiatric medications, studies addressing the medication management in youth are lacking.

When a child or adolescent in the legal system experiences a mental illness and seeks psychiatric assistance, psychoeducation is necessary. The patient and family should be educated on the causes, symptoms, course, treatment options, and treatment risks of the illness. The child should receive support in the form of active listening and motivational interviewing from a mental health provider. Family should be encouraged to participate in treatment. Adjudicated youths' parents are often not available for psychoeducation. Adjudicated youth may be in a foster home, group home, or residential treatment facility. If family are not available or are unwilling to provide support, the Department of Human Resources should address the child's mental health needs. In addition, a child advocate can be appointed by the court to facilitate treatment needs. For children who do not have consistent parents, the child's school should become involved and provide educational support in the form of special education, emotional support, or peer conflict resolution.

Therapy is the treatment of choice for many mental health disorders. Adjudicated youth are often transient. They move between family members' homes, are shuffled between foster homes, and may enter a series of residential treatment facilities before legal processes are completed. Therapy and medication management are often fractured when the living situation is inconsistent. For some adjudicated youth, consistent therapy is not an option and medication management may be easier to sustain than consistent talk therapy, although entering either course of treatment is fraught with some degree of risk. State laws vary significantly on rules for consent to medication treatment of minors and some states make additional qualifications for medication treatment of youth in juvenile justice settings.[23]

Diagnosis in child and adolescent psychiatry can be challenging for several reasons. Limited access to collateral reports from family, past psychiatric history, transient engagement in care, prevalence of undereducation and low intelligence quotient, concerns of recent substance use and prolonged withdrawal syndromes, confounding factors of trauma and psychosocial stressors, strong environmental reinforcement of exaggeration of symptoms (at best) to factitious and malingered symptoms (at worst), and the inherently stressful experience of being incarcerated at a young age increase these challenges. Several issues should be considered by prescribers before initiating medication in adjudicated youth, including:

1. How certain is the diagnosis?
2. How good is the evidence for a given medication for that diagnosis?
3. Is the youth willing to continue to take the medication, even across placements?
4. Are the parents or legal guardians in agreement with medication?
5. What are the legal parameters for consent given the age of the patient and the patient's legal status?

In short, what are the risks of treatment and nontreatment in either a correct-diagnosis or incorrect-diagnosis scenario?

SECLUSION, ISOLATION, AND SOLITARY CONFINEMENT

Seclusion and isolation may seem like similar concepts but they have distinct meanings in the context of juvenile correctional care. Seclusion and restraint are clinical interventions; isolation and solitary confinement are disciplinary measures. The National Commission on Correctional Health Care permits clinically indicated seclusion or restraint within narrow parameters but no longer allows isolation or solitary confinement.[24]

Seclusion (ie, the use of a separate physical space for a youth because of acute psychiatric symptoms that cannot be otherwise controlled through less restrictive means) is different than isolation or solitary confinement. Seclusion is a therapeutic intervention that occurs at the direction of a physician in response to psychiatric symptoms creating imminent danger to a patient or to others. The purpose of seclusion is management of agitation and prevention of harm. Seclusion is time limited, and is monitored, initiated, and ended based on clinical criteria and real-time assessment. Seclusion and therapeutic physical holds may be clinically and ethically appropriate in some limited situations in juvenile justice settings.

Any use of seclusion, restraint, isolation, or solitary confinement should occur in accordance with written and reviewed policies maintained by the facility and that are in alignment with relevant federal and state regulations, laws, and ethical standards.

In contrast, isolation and solitary confinement are disciplinary interventions that are intended to be punitive or purely a matter of security. Isolation and solitary confinement generally allow little or no contact with any people except for the facility staff and are generally not seen as being therapeutic. It is thought that such conditions can be very harmful to the wellbeing of the isolated person and raise significant ethical concerns. The American Academy of Child and Adolescent Psychiatry issued a policy statement in 2012 that permits the use of therapeutic seclusion in accordance with relevant laws and regulations but strongly discourages the use of solitary confinement or isolation and categorically disapproves of any seclusion or isolation greater than 24 hours.[25] Guidance on prohibited practices relating to isolation and solitary confinement for juveniles is an ongoing project of the American Civil Liberties Union (extensive resources available at https://www.aclu.org/report/alone-afraid).

In principle, there are cases that are clearly clinically appropriate seclusion and cases that are clearly disciplinary interventions that should not involve clinicians. Insofar as appropriate clinical, regulatory, and policy standards are followed, use of clinical seclusion and restraint may be appropriate in some circumstances. However, clinicians should be mindful that they may be asked to support or condone the correctional staff's use of isolation or other punitive or security interventions even when those interventions are clearly not clinically driven. In addition, there are, inevitably, many cases that are complex and ambiguous; clinicians are encouraged to seek consultation for any ethically challenging decision and avoid lending support to questionable practices. New resources from national professional associations have recently been released to mitigate the use of seclusion and isolation in juvenile justice settings.[26]

REFERENCES

1. US Department of Justice. Office of Justice Programs. Office of Juvenile Justice and delinquency Prevention. 2015. Available at: http://www.ojjdp.gov/ojstatbb/glossary.html. Accessed September 30, 2015.
2. Wasserman G, McReynolds L, Ko S, et al. Gender differences in psychiatric disorders at juvenile probation intake. Am J Public Health 2005;95:131–7.
3. Wasserman G, McReynolds L, Lucas D, et al. The voice DISC-IV with incarcerated male youths: prevalence of disorder. J Am Acad Child Adolesc Psychiatry 2002;41:314–21.

4. Fazel S, Doll H. Mental disorders among adolescents in juvenile detention and correctional facilities: a systemic review and metaregression analysis of 25 surveys. J Am Acad Child Adolesc Psychiatry 2008;47(9):1010–9.
5. National Center for Mental Health and Juvenile Justice. Office of Juvenile Justice and Delinquency Prevention. NCMHJJ Study.
6. Gendraue P, Goggin C. Principles of effective correctional programming. Forum on Corrections Research 1996;3:1–6.
7. Gendraue P. The principles of effective intervention with offenders. In: Harland A, editor. Choosing correctional options that work. Thousand oaks (CA): Sage Publications; 1996. p. 38–41.
8. Abram KM, Teplin LA, Charles DR, et al. Posttraumatic stress disorder and trauma in youth in juvenile detention. Arch Gen Psychiatry 2004;61(4):403–10.
9. Ford JD, Grasso DJ, Hawke J, et al. Poly-victimization among juvenile justice-involved youths. Child Abuse Negl 2013;37(10):788–800.
10. Saar MS, Epstein R, Rosenthal L, et al. The sexual abuse to prison pipeline: the girls' story. Washington, DC: Human Rights Project for Girls, Center on Poverty and Inequality at Georgetown Law, and Ms. Foundation for Women; 2015. Available at: http://rights4girls.org/wp-content/uploads/r4g/2015/02/2015_COP_sexual-abuse_layout_web-1.pdf. Accessed July 19, 2015.
11. Harris M, Fallot RD. Envisioning a trauma-informed service system: a vital paradigm shift. New Dir Ment Health Serv 2001;2001(89):3–22.
12. Jewel J, Elliff S. An investigation of the effectiveness of the Relaxation Skills Violence Prevention (RSVP) program with juvenile detainees. Crim Justice Behav 2013;40(2):203–13.
13. Perry BD, Pollard RA, Blakley TL, et al. Childhood trauma, the neurobiology of adaptation, and "use-dependent" development of the brain: how "states" become "traits"? Infant Ment Health J 1995;16(4):271–91.
14. Sherman LW, Gottfredson D, MacKenzie D, et al. Preventing crime: what works, what doesn't, what's promising? Washington, DC: Office of Justice Programs; 1997.
15. Fallot RD, Harris M. A trauma-informed approach to screening and assessment. New Dir Ment Health Serv 2001;2001(89):23–31.
16. Abram KM, Choe JY, Washburn JJ, et al. Suicidal ideation and behaviors among youths in juvenile detention. J Am Acad Child Adolesc Psychiatry 2008;47(3):291–300.
17. American Psychiatric Association. Diagnostic and statistical manual of mental disorders: DSM-5. Washington, DC: American Psychiatric Association; 2013. p. 461.
18. Kavale K, Forness S. Social skill deficits and learning disabilities: a meta-analysis. J Learn Disabil 1996;29(3):226–37.
19. Larson K. Best practices for serving court involved youth with learning, attention, and behavioral disabilities. Department of Juvenile Justice; 2002. Available at: http://cecp.air.org/juvenilejustice/docs/Promising%20and%20Preferred%20Procedures.pdf. Accessed September 30, 2015.
20. McCord J, Tremblay R. Preventing antisocial behavior: interventions from birth through adolescence. New York: Guilford Press; 1992.
21. Kazdin A. Conduct disorders in childhood and adolescence. Thousand Oaks (CA): Sage Publications; 1995.
22. Stephens TM. Social skills in the classroom. Columbus (OH): Cedars Press; 1978.
23. English A, Bass L, Boyle AD, et al. State minor consent laws: a summary. 3rd edition. Chapel Hill (NC): Center for Adolescent Health Law; 2010. Available at: http://www.cahl.org/state-minor-consent-laws-a-summary-third-edition/.

24. Standards for health services in juvenile detention and confinement facilities. Chicago: National Commission on Correctional Health Care; 2011.
25. Juvenile Justice Reform Committee. Solitary confinement of juvenile of fenders. Washington, DC: American Academy of Child and Adolescent Psychiatry; 2012.
26. Council of Juvenile Correctional Administrators toolkit: reducing the use of isolation. Braintree (MA): Council of Juvenile Correctional Administrators; 2015. Available at: http://cjca.net. Accessed July 28, 2015.

Juvenile Sex Offenders

Eileen P. Ryan, DO*

KEYWORDS

• Juvenile sex offenders • Paraphilias • Risk factors • Risk assessment
• Sex offender registries • Psychopathology • Sex offender treatment

KEY POINTS

- Sexual offending by youth is a serious problem, with approximately half of all sex offenses against children committed by individuals younger than age 18.
- Juvenile sex offenders (JSOs) comprise a heterogeneous group, and a majority of youth do not go on to develop paraphilias or to commit sex offenses during adulthood.
- As a group, JSOs are more similar to general delinquents than to adult sex offenders.
- Empirically supported risk factors for sexual reoffending in male juvenile offenders include deviant sexual interest, numerous past sexual offenses, and selection of a stranger.
- JSO risk assessments are increasingly used to inform sentencing and postsentencing decisions and hence must be performed by clinicians who possess excellent clinical skills, a thorough knowledge of normal child and adolescent development, a thorough knowledge of child and adolescent psychopathology and abnormal developmental trajectories, and an up-to-date knowledge of the research.

SCOPE OF THE PROBLEM AND DEFINITIONS

Sexual abuse by youth is neither rare nor inconsequential; victims of sexual assault suffer a variety of sequelae, including posttraumatic stress disorder (PTSD), major depression, and substance abuse.[1] Youth under the age of 18 are responsible for between 15% and 20% of all sexual offenses and up to 50% of all sexual offenses against children.[2] It has been estimated that one-third to one-half of adult sex offenders began offending as youth,[3] which can lead to the erroneous conclusion that intractable deviant sexual arousal is at the root of all sexual offending and that sexual offending youth are merely future adult sex offenders who have been caught early. As discussed throughout this article, JSOs are not just youthful adult sex offenders. They comprise a far more heterogeneous group than adult sex offenders. It is important to

Dr Ryan receives royalties from Oxford University Press.
Institute of Law, Psychiatry and Public Policy, University of Virginia School of Medicine, PO Box 800660, Charlottesville, VA 22903, USA
* Commonwealth Center for Children and Adolescents, PO Box 4000, Staunton, VA 24402.
E-mail addresses: er3h@virginia.edu; epr7857@comcast.net

Child Adolesc Psychiatric Clin N Am 25 (2016) 81–97
http://dx.doi.org/10.1016/j.chc.2015.08.010 childpsych.theclinics.com
1056-4993/16/$ – see front matter

keep in mind 2 often reiterated caveats: (1) most juveniles who commit sex offences do not go on to become sex offenders in adulthood and (2) most JSOs do not go on to develop paraphilias.

Extant research indicates that JSOs recidivate sexually at a lower rate than adult sex offenders, with most estimates of sexual reoffending ranging between 8% and 14%,[4] An examination of recidivism studies that included 11,219 JSOs with a mean follow-up period of 5 years found a mean base rate of 7.08% for sexual reoffending but a 43.4% mean base rate for general reoffending.[4] Other studies have found rates of nonsexual recidivism of 28% to 54%.[5–10] JSOs much more likely to reoffend nonsexually than sexually, and most sexual and nonsexual recidivism occurs within 3 years of release.[7,10] More recent research has focused on the ways in which JSOs are different from adolescents with histories of nonsexual offending in an effort to better identify and treat youth at risk for recidivism.[11]

The term, *sexual offender*, technically relates to an individual who has been convicted of a sexual crime and should not be assumed synonymous with any specific mental disorder(s), including paraphilias. In this article, however, the term, sex offender, is used synonymously with juveniles who engage in behaviors that meet the threshold for charges, whether or not they actually have involvement with the legal system. Management of JSOs has become more punitive over the past couple of decades. Youth as young as 10 years of age may be required to register as predatory sexual offenders for their lifetimes. Ironically, requiring convicted juveniles to be added public sex offender registries has resulted in some prosecutors being reluctant to pursue convictions and an increase in plea bargain deals, including sex offense charges amended to nonsexual charges and lower severity charges.[12] Additionally, it seems that juvenile registration has little deterrent effect on behavior considered to be sexual offenses.[13]

WHAT CAUSES JUVENILE SEXUAL OFFENDING?

There are undoubtedly a variety of etiologies of sexual offending. Biological, familial, societal, and developmental factors have all been postulated as playing a role in the onset and continuation of sexual offending. As discussed in this article, JSOs are a varied group, and the onset of sexual offending in a specific person is as unique as the individual. A comprehensive theoretic framework regarding the cause of sexual offending is lacking. Descriptive studies categorize JSOs into 3 groups: (1) those with underlying sexual deviation, (2) those with a general antisocial orientation, and (3) those with traits that indicate more general psychopathology.[14] Although numerous theories regarding the etiology of sexual offending in adults have been proposed,[15–17] there is no generally accepted theory regarding the cause of sexual offending in youth. Several etiologic factors have received empirical and clinical interest, however, including a history of maltreatment, especially sexual abuse; exposure to pornography; and exposure to aggressive role models.[18]

Ryan and colleagues[19] proposed a model of sexual offending that begins with a negative sense of self, in which vulnerable children and adolescents protect themselves from what they predict will be negative and hurtful interaction by social withdrawal and isolation. They retreat into fantasy to compensate for feelings of powerlessness and helplessness. When sexual offending occurs, there is a further increase in negative emotions and self-image and thoughts of rejection, establishing a destructive repetitive cycle. In the Marshall and Barbaree model,[20–22] children learn that they are more successful at getting their parents' or caretakers' attention by being disruptive, which in turn leads to caretakers adopting an aggressive, coercive, and manipulative parenting style, which limits children's experiences of prosocial, nurturing interactions. When children enter school, they are less likely to successfully manage impulses and negotiate positive, healthy relationships with peers or teachers. These relationship problems lead to a negative self-image and lack of confidence. From there, what the investigators call a "syndrome of social disability" develops, with the emergence and consolidation of sexually abusive behavior as part of a larger framework of antisocial or delinquent behavior. This theoretic model suggests that understanding and tackling those aspects of the family that promote criminal behavior are critical in the development of a treatment plan.

Becker and Kaplan[23,24] proposed that the first sex offense results from a combination of individual characteristics, including a lack of social skills, a history of nonsexual deviance, family variables, and social-environmental variables, such as social isolation and antisocial behavior. After the first sex offenses, youth may pursue 3 possible paths: (1) a dead end, in which there are no further crimes; (2) a delinquency path, in which the juvenile engages in continued sexual offending and in general nonsexual offenses and deviant behaviors; and (3) a sexual interest path, in which the juvenile continues to commit sexual offenses and develops a paraphilia. Shaw and Antia[25] identified 4 types of JSOs: (1) youth with true paraphilias, (2) youth with strong antisocial personality traits, (3) youth compromised by a neurologic disorder (mental retardation, autistic spectrum disorder, and so forth), and (4) youth with impaired social skills who turn to younger children for sexual gratification. Hunter and colleagues[26] noted that male adolescents who offended against prepubescent children had greater deficits in psychosocial functioning, engaged in less aggression during the offense, and were more likely to offend against relatives. Physical abuse by a father or stepfather and exposure to violence against girls and women were found associated with higher levels of comorbid anxiety and depression among youthful sex offenders. Noncoercive childhood sexual abuse by a male nonrelative was found associated with sexual offending against a male child.

RISK FACTORS FOR JUVENILE SEXUAL OFFENDING

Long before research on JSOs, deviant sexual arousal was noted in adult male sex offenders. Deviant sexual interest is clearly a risk factor for recidivism in adults, with studies of male sexual offenders indicating that most of the participants had developed deviant arousal in adolescence. Abel and colleagues[27,28] reported that 42% of adults diagnosed with paraphilias reported deviant sexual arousal by 15 years of age and 57% by age 19.

In the past, youth who engaged in sexually offensive conduct were frequently perceived as engaging in sexual experimentation than criminal behavior. Although some adolescents and children are sexually reactive and engage in sexually offensive behavior as part of a phase related to inappropriate sexual exploration, this should not be automatically assumed. A minority of adolescents do have deviant sexual arousal patterns, have had prior victims, and are beginning a pattern of behavior that is similar to that of adult paraphilic sexual offenders.[9,29] Recent research has attempted to focus on better understanding and improved identification of youth who may be at higher risk for adult sex offending.

According to the *Diagnostic and Statistical Manual of Mental Disorders* (Fifth Edition),[30] paraphilias are characterized by "any intense and persistent sexual interest other than sexual interest in genital stimulation or preparatory fondling with phenotypically normal, physically mature, consenting human partners." (See **Box 1** for a brief description of individual paraphilias.) To qualify for the diagnosis of a paraphilia, these

Box 1
Paraphilias

Pedophilia

Recurrent, intense sexually arousing fantasies, sexual urges, or behaviors involving sexual activity with prepubescent children (usually age 13 years or younger) over a period of ≥6 months. The individual is age ≥16 and ≥5 years older than the child. The individual has acted on the urges or they cause significant distress or interpersonal difficulty.

Voyeurism

Recurrent, intense sexual arousal over a period ≥6 months, as manifested by fantasies, urges, or behaviors from observing an unsuspecting person who is naked, in the process of disrobing, or engaging in sexual activity. The individual has acted on the urges or they cause significant distress or social or occupational difficulty.

Exhibitionism

Recurrent, intense sexual arousal, over a period ≥6 months, from the exposure of one's genitals to an unsuspecting person, as manifested by fantasies, urges, or behaviors. The individual has acted on the urges or they cause significant distress or social or occupational difficulty.

Frotteurism

Recurrent and intense sexual arousal from touching or rubbing up against a nonconsenting person, as manifested by fantasies, urges, or behaviors, over a period ≥6 months. The individual has acted on the urges or they cause significant distress or social or occupational difficulty.

Sexual masochism

Recurrent, intense sexual arousal from being humiliated, beaten, bound, or otherwise made to suffer, over a period ≥6 months, as manifested by fantasies, urges, or behaviors. The individual has acted on the urges or they cause significant distress or social or occupational difficulty.

Sexual sadism

Recurrent, intense sexual arousal from the physical or psychological suffering of another person, as manifested by fantasies, urges, or behaviors, over a period ≥6 months, The individual has acted on the urges or they cause significant distress or social or occupational difficulty.

Fetishism

Recurrent, intense sexual arousal from either the use of nonliving objects or a highly specific focus on nongenital body parts, as manifested by fantasies, urges, or behaviors, over a period of ≥6 months, causing significant distress or impairment in social or occupational functioning.

Transvestism

Recurrent, intense sexual arousal from cross-dressing, as manifested by fantasies, urges, or behaviors, over a period of ≥6 months, with significant distress or impairment in social or occupational functioning.

Zoophilia

Recurrent, intense sexual arousal involving animals as manifested by fantasies, urges, or behaviors, over a period of ≥6 months, with significant distress or impairment in social or occupational functioning.

Coprohilia

Recurrent, intense sexual arousal from feces as manifested by fantasies, urges, or behaviors, over a period of ≥6 months, with significant distress or impairment in social or occupational functioning.

Urophilia

Recurrent, intense sexual arousal from urine, as manifested by fantasies, urges, or behaviors, over a period of ≥6 months, with significant distress or impairment in social or occupational functioning.

Necrophilia

Recurrent, intense sexual arousal from corpses, as manifested by fantasies, urges, or behaviors, over a period of ≥6 months, with significant distress or impairment in social or occupational functioning.

Klismaphilia

Recurrent, intense sexual arousal from enemas, as manifested by fantasies, urges, or behaviors, over a period of ≥6 months, with significant distress or impairment in social or occupational functioning.

Telephone scatologia

Recurrent, intense sexual arousal from making obscene phone calls, as manifested by fantasies, urges, or behaviors, over a period of ≥6 months, with significant distress or impairment in social or occupational functioning.

Data from American Psychiatric Association. Diagnostic and statistical manual of mental disorders (DSM-5). 5th edition. Washington, DC: American Psychiatric Association; 2013.

behaviors must have occurred for at least 6 months and have caused distress or impairment that impedes social, occupational, or other important areas of functioning. Deviant sexual arousal is a critical component of any paraphilia.

Identifying and targeting paraphilias in adult sex offenders are critical in evaluation and treatment planning. Adults with paraphilias are at increased risk for sexual reoffending.[31–34] Most juveniles who engage in sexually offensive behavior do not go on to develop a paraphilia, but some will.[27] Identifying those adolescents at risk for developing paraphilias and reoffending sexually is one of the most vexing of challenges. The adult literature is not terribly helpful when applied to juveniles. As an example, consider the use of phallometric testing, or penile plethysmography, considered the gold standard of objective measurement of sexual arousal in men based on extensive research on its reliability and validity.[35] Among adult sex offenders, deviant sexual arousal as measured by penile plethysmography has been noted the most predictive factor for sexual reoffending among pedophilic adult sex offenders[32]; however, in adolescents the results are mixed.[36] Gretton and colleagues[37] reported no association between repeated sexual offending and deviant sexual arousal in JSOs as measured by phallometric assessment in an outpatient sample of 220 male juvenile offenders; however, they did find that juveniles with both elevated psychopathy and deviant sexual arousal were at increased risk for general recidivism. A more recent study considered the discriminative and predictive validity of the penile plethysmography in a sample of 132 male adolescent sex offenders admitted to a sex offender treatment program. The subjects were assessed pretreatment and post-treatment, under an "arouse" condition (subjects allowed themselves to become aroused) and a "suppress" condition (subjects attempted to suppress or control their arousal). Post-treatment arousal and inability to suppress arousal to male and female children were significantly related to sexual offense recidivism.[38]

Risk assessments are increasingly used to inform decisions regarding sentencing and postsentencing conditions, including community notification and registration, treatment needs, and supervision requirements. A risk assessment is, therefore, a high-stakes evaluation, and evaluators must possess a thorough and up-to-date knowledge of the ever-expanding research on juveniles as well as excellent clinical skills and adequate time to perform an evaluation thoroughly.

Vignette 1

Joe is a 14-year-old boy with a full-scale IQ of 72 and a history of anxiety, depression, ADHD, and sexual abuse by a neighborhood adolescent, who revealed during a therapy session that he was "playing" with his 6-year-old sister while minding her when his single-parent mother was working during the evenings. His description of the "play" revealed mutual fondling, with clothes off, which began several months ago when he was bathing his sister prior to her bedtime and progressed to intercourse. His therapist, as a mandated reporter, informed child protective services. Joe was subsequently charged with a sexual felony, placed in a juvenile detention center, and quickly transferred from juvenile to adult court. A psychosexual evaluation did not indicate evidence of deviant sexual arousal. Joe was found incompetent to stand trial and spent about 9 months being restored to competency in the detention center. At age 16, Joe ultimately pleaded guilty in a deal that allowed him to serve his sentence in juvenile corrections, where he was remanded until age 21, and placed on the adult sexual offender registry for life.

Vignette 2

Robbie is a 15-year-old boy who was in the custody of social services for 3 months, when he was taken into custody after several boys and girls, ages 4 to 8, revealed to their parents that Robbie has fondled them and forced them to masturbate him at a church camp. A police examination of the biological family's computer revealed numerous downloaded images of sexual acts involving very young children; however, it could not be proved that Robbie was the individual who downloaded the images, and his father, who denied knowing about the images, was recently incarcerated for sexually abusing a 12-year-old cousin. Robbie denies a history of sexual abuse or physical abuse but has witnessed domestic abuse. His mother was arrested for prostitution several months ago, but the charges were dropped. Robbie has several friends and is a good student and on the high school track team. He denies that he is gay but does not have a girlfriend, indicating that he is too young to be interested in girls.

- *These 2 cases reveal the importance of thorough clinical evaluation and risk assessment as well as a knowledge of empirically validated risk factors for reoffending. The fact that penetration was involved in Joe's case does not increase his risk for sexual recidivism. A risk assessment evaluation may have revealed that the convergence of cognitive limitations, social isolation and poor social skills, poor supervision, and opportunity were critical risk factors for the initiation of Joe's abuse of his sister. Although extant research indicates that a history of sexual abuse may be a risk factor for the initiation of sexual abuse, especially in combination with other risk factors, it is not a risk factor for sexual recidivism.*
- *Joe's ultimate fate reveals the reality of overcharging youth who have committed sexual offenses and are at low risk for sexual recidivism—delayed or minimal treatment and the imposition of long-standing or even lifelong obstacles to employment (felony criminal record and sex offender registration) and adult independence in a youth who already has a variety of vulnerabilities.*

- *Robbie, despite his intelligence and involvement in prosocial activities, presents with several risk factors for sexual reoffending, most importantly multiple stranger victims, and several red flags for possible deviant sexual arousal that should be carefully assessed, including probable exposure to child pornography, even if he did not download the images; exposure to parental sexuality and violence; and an apparent lack of sexual interest in same-age peers.*
- *At first glance, Robbie's risk for sexual reoffending seems much higher than Joe. If a thorough sex offender risk assessment bears that out, he should receive sex offender–specific treatment in a residential facility.*

Worling and Langstrom[39] divided risk factors for sexual recidivism into 4 categories: supported, promising, probable, and unlikely. Empirically supported risk factors for recidivism include deviant sexual interest, attitudes supportive of sexual offending, numerous past sexual offenses, selection of a stranger, lack of intimate peer relationships or social isolation, high-stress family life, problematic parent-offender relationships, and incomplete sex offender treatment. Risk factors are difficult to measure, however, and have not been validated as predictive of recidivism in any sex offender risk assessment instrument. Also, some of the risk factors associated with reoffense are nonspecific and associated not only with nonsexual delinquency but also with compromised mental health in general.

Christiansen and Vincent[40] studied 39,248 adjudicated juvenile sexual and nonsexual offenders ages 7 to 18 years in Maricopa County, Arizona. The sexual reoffense rate was 4.2%, and the reoffense rate for nonsexual crimes was 40.96%, reflecting the trend noted in other studies; that is, as a group JSOs are far more likely to recidivate nonsexually than sexually. The fact that only 1.77% of the sample had any adjudicated sex offense illustrates the problem that extremely low base rates presents in the prediction of both juvenile sexual offending generally and reoffending in particular. The extremely low base rate makes development of an instrument that effectively and specifically identifies only those juveniles at risk for reoffending sexually very difficult. In this study, among the strongest predictors of sexual recidivism were prior nonsexual offending, prior sexual offending, hands-off offending, offending against a child, not attending school, and younger school grade/age at the time of the initial offense.[40]

Recent research has focused on distinctions between the larger generalist group and much smaller group of specialist JSOs. Seto and Lalumière[11] conducted a meta-analysis of 59 studies comparing male adolescent sex offenders (N = 3855) with adolescent offenders who had not committed sexual offenses (N = 13,393) on a variety of variables, including conduct problems and criminal involvement, maltreatment and exposure to violence, substance abuse, family and interpersonal problems, sexuality, and psychopathology. The results of their meta-analysis revealed that on many variables the 2 groups did not differ, including antisocial personality traits, attitudes, and beliefs; early conduct problems; intelligence; social problems; and general psychopathology. Adolescent sex offenders had a less extensive criminal history, less substance abuse, and fewer delinquent friends. Adolescent sex offenders also differed from their generalist peers with respect to variables related to psychosexual development and maltreatment history; they were much more likely to have been sexually abused and more likely to have been physically and emotionally abused. Adolescent sex offenders were more likely to have had early exposure to sex or pornography, exposure to sexual violence within the family, and atypical sexual interests (eg, sexual fantasies involving young children or coerced sex). The largest differences found were with respect to atypical sexual interests and sexual abuse history. The investigators suggested that although adolescent sex offenders and general delinquents share many of the same risk factors for offending, to understand why an adolescent commits a sex offense rather than a nonsexual offense, special factors, including a history of sexual abuse, exposure to sex or pornography, and atypical sexual interests, need to be considered.[41]

PSYCHIATRIC EVALUATION AND PSYCHOPATHOLOGY

Several studies of adult sex offenders with paraphilic and nonparaphilic deviant behavior have indicated high rates of comorbid psychiatric disorders, especially mood, anxiety, substance abuse, and personality disorders.[42–45] The few studies of comorbidity in adolescent sex offenders indicate a high incidence of diverse psychiatric pathology. Sex offending is a behavior, however, not a diagnosis, and as such has numerous causes and manifestations.[46] Psychiatric evaluation disconnected from risk assessment is of limited utility. Psychiatric disorders, with the infrequent exceptions of mania and psychosis, do not "cause" sexual offending; however, ignoring psychiatric comorbidity in offenders can seriously compromise the efficacy of structured sex offender treatment. There are few studies of psychopathology among JSOs. A study that identified 34 JSOs broken out of a sample of 242 chronic violent juvenile offenders found few characteristics associated with conduct disorder, with fewer drug and alcohol problems and less frequent involvement in gangs. These JSOs were more likely to have been raised in families with spousal violence, physical abuse, and sexual abuse. They were more sexually and socially isolated, with stronger beliefs in law and order but fewer internal controls on their behavior.[47] Another study of psychopathology in 58 male sex offenders ages 13 to 18 referred for outpatient evaluation and treatment found conduct disorder the most prevalent diagnosis (48%), with 8.3% meeting criteria for alcohol abuse, 10.3% for both alcohol and cannabis abuse, 8.6% for adjustment disorder with depressed mood, 6.9% for attention-deficit/hyperactivity disorder (ADHD), and 5.2% for social phobia. No diagnosis was found in 19.2%, with the investigators hypothesizing that the lack of more severe psychopathology was related to the fact that more severely affected sexual offenders were referred to hospital or residential programs.[48]

Personality pathology in sexually offending youth has received research attention, but findings are often contradictory, which is not surprising, given the heterogeneity of this population. Psychopathy, a multidimensional construct or personality style, encompasses interpersonal (manipulative or grandiose), affective (callous or shallow), lifestyle (impulsive or stimulation seeking), and antisocial (criminal orientation) features and is of interest because of its robust association with general and violent crime.[49] Psychopathy has been noted in several studies to predict general and sexual recidivism in adolescent boys.[37,50] There is controversy around the stability of psychopathic traits into adulthood and concerns regarding the potential misuse of the diagnosis to divert adolescents into correctional facilities rather than into treatment.[51] Also, psychopathy does not seem a useful predictor of violent or nonviolent recidivism in girls.[52]

Although there is limited research on psychopathology in JSOs specifically, research over the past 10 to 15 years on delinquent youth generally (which includes sex offenders) indicates that the prevalence of mental illness is much higher in incarcerated youth than in the general adolescent population. A meta-analysis of the research on the prevalence of mental disorders among incarcerated juveniles in short-term detention and longer-term correctional facilities involving 13,778 boys and 2972 girls (ranging from 10 to 19 years, with a mean age 15.6 years)[53] found that among boys, 3.3% were diagnosed with psychosis, 10.6% with major depression, 11.7% with ADHD, and 52.8% with conduct disorder. Among the girls, 2.7% were diagnosed with psychosis, 29.2% with major depression, 18.5% with ADHD, and 52.8% with conduct disorder. The prevalence of major depression found in delinquent girls (29.2%) is considerably higher than found in adult female prison populations (12%).[54]

In a randomly selected sample of 1172 male and 657 female detainees studied over 6 months,[55] approximately half had substance use disorders, with 21% having 2 or more disorders. Of those youth with any substance use disorder, approximately 50% also had an alcohol use disorder.

Trauma and PTSD are more prevalent among detained youth than in community samples, with 83% of boys and 84% of girls among 898 youth ages 10 to 18 years reporting at least 1 traumatic experience, and 11% of the sample meeting criteria for PTSD with the past year.[56,57] Among youth with PTSD, comorbidity was the rule rather than the exception with 93% having at least 1 and 54% having 2 or more comorbid psychiatric disorders (mood, anxiety, or behavioral or substance abuse disorders), and 11% having 4 comorbid disorders. Among 1829 newly detained youth ages 10 to 18 years, more than one-third of detainees and approximately one-half of the girls felt hopeless and had thoughts of death in the 6 months prior to detention, with 10% considering suicide and 10% having made a suicide attempt in the past 6 months.[58]

FEMALE JUVENILE SEX OFFENDERS

Adolescent female sex offenders are an understudied group for 2 reasons: (1) the small numbers of girls who commit sexual offenses and (2) the low rates of sexual recidivism for female sex offenders. It has been estimated that only approximately 5% to 10 % of all juvenile sex offenses are committed by female adolescents,[59,60] and a meta-analysis of 10 studies of the recidivism rates of female adolescents who had committed sex offenses with an average follow-up of 6.5 years found that less than 3% recidivated.[61]

A study of female adolescent sex offenders in Washington state[62] showed that risk factors for general recidivism were least common in female adolescents who had committed a felony sexual offense against a younger child, and these girls had fewer problems in the domains of school, family, and friends than did adolescent girls who had committed a misdemeanor sexual offense or a felony sexual offense with a peer victim. Girls who had committed a felony offense against a peer or a misdemeanor sexual offense more closely resembled female adolescent nonsexual offenders. They demonstrated a high prevalence for risk factors for general (nonsexual) recidivism, such as severe behavior problems in school, truancy, parental alcohol and mental health problems, running away, out-of-home placements, poor parental control, and delinquent friends. There were no differences in mental health problems. These findings mirror results from studies of adolescent male sex offenders, in that those adolescents who abused children were less similar to nonsexual offending delinquents than peer abusers and had a low prevalence of risk factors for general recidivism. In another study using the same cohort, sexual victimization by a nonrelative was the only characteristic that distinguished girls who had committed sexual offenses from adolescent male sex offenders and adolescent female nonsexual violent offenders.[63]

TESTING AND USE OF STRUCTURED INSTRUMENTS

In the assessment of adult sex offenders, actuarial measures, such as the Static-99 and Static-2002, which are supported by more than 60 validity studies, are a mainstay of evaluation[64,65] The evaluation of sexually offending youth requires far more than psychological assessment instruments, and at present there is no instrument or measure that predicts sexual offending or recidivism. This is not surprising given that the base rate of sexual recidivism is low and most juvenile sexual offenders are more similar to other delinquents than to adult sex offenders and are more likely to commit a nonsexual offense than a sexual offense. The outcome of sexual recidivism is a highly unusual one, and it is extremely difficult to develop an actuarial instrument that is able to predict such an unusual outcome.

The 3 instruments most frequently used in JSO evaluations are the Juvenile Sex Offender Assessment Protocol-II (J-SOAP-II), the Estimate of Risk of Adolescent Sexual Offense Recidivism (ERASOR), and the Psychopathy Checklist: Youth Version (PCL:YV). The J-SOAP-II, an empirically informed guide designed for use in boys ages 12 to 18 for the assessment of risk factors associated with sexual and violent offending, is one of the most commonly instruments in the United States.[66] Results are mixed, however, with for the instrument as a whole or for individual subscales to predict sexual or nonsexual recidivism.[67] Recent studies indicate that it can be a useful adjunct to assessment, but additional risk assessment is necessary for a thorough evaluation.[68]

Results for the ERASOR,[69] which has the stated purpose of only predicting sexual recidivism, are likewise equivocal.[67] A recent meta-analysis of risk assessment instruments found that tools specifically designed for adolescents did not outperform the Static-99, which was developed for adult sex offenders and is not recommended for use in juveniles. The investigators note, however, that the overlap in risk factors for adolescent and adult offending as well as the effect size for the Static-99 likely contributed to the findings.[70]

The PCL:YV, although a strong predictor of general recidivism, does not predict sexual recidivism,[67] although in 1 study an extremely high (greater than 34) score on the PCL:YV was predictive of sexual recidivism.[71]

TREATMENT

Given the heterogeneity of JSOs, a one-size-fits-all approach to treatment is ill advised, and treatment should be tailored to individual youths and to the risk factors uncovered from a comprehensive psychiatric evaluation and forensic risk assessment. Treatment should target dynamic risk factors as well as protective factors identified in evaluation and risk assessment, and any treatment program, whether it is an outpatient community treatment program or a residential program, should have procedures in place for ongoing assessment of dynamic risk factors. Without an understanding of the risk factors specific to the individual youth and to the offense, it is impossible to assess the significance and impact of those factors to the youth and the offense and plan for treatment. For example, if depression had little to do with the offense, treating depression in the JSO with paraphilic arousal, although a clinical and moral imperative, does little to minimize the risk of reoffending either generally or sexually. It is the deviant sexual arousal that presents the most risk of sexual reoffending and that needs to be specifically addressed in treatment.

Although additional research on empirically validated treatment approaches for sexually offending youth is sorely needed, there are interventions that have some demonstrated efficacy, but adopting them has been slow. The prevailing approach used in outpatient and residential treatments is a combination of cognitive behavioral group therapy and relapse prevention.[72] A 20-year prospective follow-up study found that the base rates for sexual (9%), nonsexual violent (22%), nonviolent (28%), and general reoffending (38%) were significantly lower for youth who participated in specialized treatment versus a comparison group (with 21%, 39%, 52%, and 57% base rates, respectively).[73]

All adjudicated JSOs should be engaged in sex-offender specific treatment, including individualized sex-offender specific services to those youth returning to the community from residential placement. This transition from residential treatment (whether court-ordered in a private facility or in a juvenile correctional program) is where treatment planning and execution frequently falls apart, leaving both the juvenile and community vulnerable. Hunter developed guidelines for making level-of-care determinations on JSOs for the Virginia Department of Juvenile Justice, with the intention of complementing, not replacing, formal clinical and risk assessment.[74] He developed clinical profiles for youth at "low," "moderate," and "high" risks of reoffending based on a youth's sexual offenses and criminal history, psychosexual characteristics, peer affiliations and family characteristics, and past response to treatment. Low risk youth were characterized as those that had engaged in nonviolent, time-limited (1 to 2 times) sexual behaviors that were relatively noninvasive and noncoercive and typically exploratory and opportunistic (eg, fondling of younger siblings or children for whom the offender was babysitting). These low-risk offenders had no or minimal criminal histories and age-appropriate sexual interests and were without a history of prior sexual offending or inappropriate sexual behavior. Their families were not highly dysfunctional. The low-risk offender is appropriate for community-based care and probation. Moderate-risk offenders' sexual offending began in adolescence and they engaged in sexual offenses that involved trickery or mild physical or verbal coercion; however, the offenses were nonviolent in nature. The offense may have involved fondling, exposure, oral sex, or attempted vaginal or anal intercourse. The victims were not strangers, and typically younger siblings or family members or acquaintances. The moderate-risk offenders come from moderately dysfunctional families and have a history of maltreatment or exposure to antisocial behavior; parents may minimize the significance of the adolescent's behavior and/or feel overwhelmed and unable to cope. In Hunter's guidelines, moderate-risk youth are seen as requiring more intensive, wrap-around community-based services and court supervision. High-risk offenders were characterized as those who engage in planned sexual offenses that involved the use of threats, deception, or physical force and involved vaginal or anal penetration, with multiple incidents extending over a period of time. Offenders with stranger victims were placed in this category. A history of nonsexual or sexual offenses of a highly aggressive nature is present. These youth show evidence of deviant sexual interests or antisocial personality traits, and offending against younger children reflects pedophilic interests. Offending against same-age peers or adults reflects endorsement of rape myths and fantasy. The youth does not learn from past experiences and repeats problematic behavior in multiple environments. The family system is typically moderately to severely dysfunctional. The high-risk offender generally required residential treatment (in a juvenile justice facility or court-ordered) with 24-hour supervision and care.

For juveniles identified as a generalist offenders, proved treatments targeting delinquency are warranted, such multisystemic therapy (MST), functional family therapy, or multidimensional family therapy. For specialist offenders, treatments such as cognitive behavioral therapy focusing on management of atypical and deviant sexual arousal as well as sexual preoccupations may be beneficial. Even in the adult literature, treatment outcome studies must be interpreted cautiously, given their methodological limitations. A meta-analysis by Hanson and colleagues[75] examining treatment efficacy with adult male offenders found that cognitive behavioral therapy significantly decreased sexual recidivism compared with no treatment (12% sexual recidivism vs 17% without treatment). In a 20-year follow-up of adolescents who received specialized community-based treatment, Worling and colleagues[73] found that those who participated in specialized treatment, the Sexual Abuse: Family Education and Treatment Program, were significantly less likely than those in a comparison group to receive subsequent charges for sexual (9% vs 21%), nonsexual violent (22% vs 39%), and nonviolent crimes (28% vs 52%). The program contains a major family component, as do other successful programs targeting this population.[76–78]

A 2-year follow-up of a randomized effectiveness trial evaluating MST supported the ability of MST to sustain positive changes among juvenile sexual offenders. Although sexual recidivism was too low to conduct statistical analysis, there was no between-groups difference with respect to rearrests for nonsexual offenses.[78]

A small percentage of juvenile substance users requires residential treatment. One of the major drawbacks of residential treatment is that their distance from youths' families makes frequent necessary family work difficult if not impossible. It is this author's opinion that the unfortunate practice noted in recent years of conducting family work by phone (which is billable as family therapy) is a poor substitute for the type of intensive family engagement and therapy that most of these youths' families require. It is known that too much intervention with nonsexually offending juveniles does little good and may actually have negative effects. If the goal is to decrease subsequent delinquent and criminal behavior, juvenile offenders with low risk for reoffending should be diverted from the juvenile justice system. Subjecting delinquents to punishments and interventions beyond what is necessary actually increases the risk of recidivism.[79]

Pharmacologic Treatment

JSOs may also have co-occurring psychiatric disorders, especially mood and anxiety disorders as well as ADHD for which pharmacologic treatment is indicated. Unless their psychiatric disorders are appropriately treated, afflicted youth may be unable to participate fully in sex offender treatment. Unfortunately, the quality of the evidence base for pharmacologic treatments of sexual offending, which is almost entirely for adults, is poor. The World Federation of Societies of Biological Psychiatry developed guidelines on the biological treatment of adults with paraphilias.[80] There is even less research available to guide decision making in the pharmacologic treatment of adolescents with paraphilias. The gold standard of demonstrating pharmacologic efficacy is the randomized, double blind, placebo-controlled trial. Although selective serotonin reuptake inhibitors (SSRIs) have enjoyed widespread use with the goal of decreasing sexual obsessions and compulsive sexual behavior in both adults and youth, there are no randomized placebo-controlled studies of their use in paraphilias. Because of their methodological limitations, a critical analysis of all published studies concluded that there was only minimal research evidence to support their efficacy.[80] Because of their ease of use and favorable side-effect profile (including the typically undesired side effect of decreased libido), however, SSRIs are the most frequently used medication used targeting sexual behavior in sexually offending juveniles. The similarities between obsessive-compulsive disorder and paraphilic and nonparaphilic sexual disorders have been noted by Bradford and others.[81–83] Despite the frequency with which SSRIs are used in the juvenile offender population, especially targeting deviant arousal, there are only 2 open label trials an SSRI (fluoxetine) targeting paraphilic behavior described in the literature, both with a positive response.[84,85]

A minority of adolescent sex offenders do have deviant sexual arousal/paraphilias and have reoffended repeatedly. Treatment with hormonal agents, such as medroxyprogesterone acetate and luteinizing hormone-releasing hormone, however, frequently used in adult repeat offenders, is rarely used with adolescents in the United States secondary to their side-effect profiles and as-yet unknown potential sequelae in adolescents who are still developing. For a more in-depth discussion of hormonal agents, readers are referred to the review of biological therapies by Ryan.[86]

REFERENCES

1. Heim C, Shugart M, Craighead WE, et al. Neurobiological and psychiatric consequences of child abuse and neglect. Dev Psychobiol 2010;52(7):671–90.
2. Zolendek MA, Abel GG, Northey WF, et al. Self-reported behaviors of juvenile sexual offenders. Prev Res 2002;9(4):14–6.
3. Prentky R, Harris B, Frizzel K, et al. An actuarial procedure for assessing risk in juvneile sex offenders. Sex Abuse 2000;12(2):71–93.
4. Caldwell MF. Study characteristics and recidivism base rates in juvenile sex offender recidivism. Int J Offender Ther Comp Criminol 2010;54(2):197–212.
5. Caldwell MF. What we do not know about juvenile sexual reoffense risk. Child Maltreat 2002;7(4):291–302.
6. Vandiver DM. A prospective analysis of juvenile male sex offenders: characteristics and recidivism rates as adults. J Interpers Violence 2006;21(5):673–88.
7. Waite D, Keller A, McGarvey EL, et al. Juvenile sex offender re-arrest rates for sexual, violent nonsexual and property crimes: a 10-year follow-up. Sex Abuse 2005;17(3):313–31.
8. Becker J, Cunningham-Rathier J, Kaplan M. Adolescent sex offenders. J Interpers Violence 1986;1:431–5.
9. Fehrenbach PA, Smith W, Monastersky C, et al. Adolescent sexual offenders: offender and offense characteristics. Am J Orthopsychiatry 1986;56(2):225–33.
10. Caldwell MF. Sexual offense adjudication and sexual recidivism among juvenile offenders. Sex Abuse 2007;19(2):107–13.
11. Seto MC, Lalumière ML. What is so special about male adolescent sexual offending? A review and test of explanations through meta-analysis. Psychol Bull 2010; 136(4):526–75.
12. Letourneau EJ, Armstrong KS, Bandyopadhyay D, et al. Sex offender registration and notification policy increases juvenile plea bargains. Sex Abuse 2013;25(2): 189–207.
13. Stevenson MC, Najdowski CJ, Wiley TR. Knowledge of juvenile sex offender registration laws predicts adolescent sexual behavior. J Child Sex Abus 2013; 22(1):103–18.
14. O'Shaughnessy RJ. Violent adolescent sexual offenders. Child Adolesc Psychiatr Clin N Am 2002;11(4):749–65.
15. Lanyon RI. Scientific status of the concept of continuing emotional propensity for sexually aberrant acts. J Am Acad Psychiatry Law 1997;25(1):59–67.
16. Stinson JD, Becker JV, Sales BD. Self-regulation and the etiology of sexual deviance: evaluating causal theory. Violence Vict 2008;23(1):35–51.
17. Whitaker DJ, Le B, Karl Hanson R, et al. Risk factors for the perpetration of child sexual abuse: a review and meta-analysis. Child Abuse Negl 2008;32(5):529–48.
18. Becker JV, Hunter JA. Understanding and treating child and juvenile sex offenders. In: Ollendick TH, Prinz RJ, editors. Advances in clinical child psychology, vol. 1. New York: Plenum Press; 1997. 177-197.
19. Ryan G, Lane S, Davis J, et al. Juvenile sex offenders: development and correction. Child Abuse Negl 1987;11(3):385–95.

20. Barbaree HE, Marshall WL, McCormick J. The development of sexually deviant behaviour among adolescents and its implications for prevention and treatment. Irish J Psychol 1998;19(1):1–31.
21. Marshall WL, Barbaree HE. An integrated theory of the origins of sexual offending. In: Marshall WL, Laws DR, Barbaree HE, editors. Handbook of sexual assault: issues, theories, and treatment of the offender. New York: Plenum Press; 1990. p. 257–75.
22. Marshall WL, Marshall L. The origins of sexual offending. Trauma Violence Abuse 2000;1:250–63.
23. Becker JV, Kaplan MS. The assessment of juvenile sex offenders. In: Prinz RJ, editor. Advances in behavioral assessment in children and families, vol. 4. Greenwich (CT): JAI Press; 1988. p. 97–118.
24. Becker JV, Hicks SJ. Juvenile sexual offenders: characteristics, interventions, and policy issues. Ann N Y Acad Sci 2003;989:397–410 [discussion: 441–5].
25. Shaw JA, Antia DK. Sexually aggressive youth. In: Benedek EP, Ash P, Scott CL, editors. Principles and practice of child and adolescent forensic mental health. 2nd edition. Arlington (VA): American Psychiatric Publishing; 2009. p. 389–401.
26. Hunter JA, Figueredo AJ, Malamuth NM, et al. Juvenile sex offenders: toward the development of a typology. Sex Abuse 2003;15(1):27–48.
27. Abel GG, Coffey L, Osborn CA. Sexual arousal patterns: normal and deviant. Psychiatr Clin North Am 2008;31(4):643–55.
28. Abel GG, Jordan A, Rouleau JL, et al. Use of visual reaction time to assess male adolescents who molest children. Sex Abuse 2004;16(3):255–65.
29. Becker JV, Hunter JA, Stein RM, et al. Factors associated with erection in adolescent sex offenders. J Psychopathol Behav Assess 1989;11:353–62.
30. American Psychiatric Association. Diagnostic and statistical manual of mental disorders (DSM-5). 5th edition. Washington, DC: American Psychiatric Press; 2013.
31. Abracen J, Mailloux DL, Serin RC, et al. A model for the assessment of static and dynamic factors in sexual offenders. J Sex Res 2004;41(4):321–8.
32. Hanson RK, Bussiere MT. Predicting relapse: a meta-analysis of sexual offender recidivism studies. J Consult Clin Psychol 1998;66(2):348–62.
33. Prentky RA, Lee AFS, Knight RA, et al. Recidivism rates among child molesters and rapists: a methodological analysis. Law Hum Behav 1997;21(6):635–59.
34. Prentky RA, Knight RA, Lee AF. Risk factors associated with recidivism among extrafamilial child molesters. J Consult Clin Psychol 1997;65(1):141–9.
35. Murphy L, Ranger R, Stewart H, et al. Assessment of problematic sexual interests with the penile plethysmograph: an overview of assessment laboratories. Curr Psychiatry Rep 2015;17(29):1–5.
36. Mackaronis JE, Byrne PM, Strassberg DS. Assessing sexual interest in adolescents who have sexually offended. Sex Abuse 2014. [Epub ahead of print].
37. Gretton HM, McBride M, Hare RD, et al. Psychopathy and recidivism in adolescent sex offenders. Crim Justice Behav 2001;28:427–49.
38. Clift RJ, Rajlic G, Gretton HM. Discriminative and predictive validity of the penile plethysmograph in adolescent sex offenders. Sex Abuse 2009;21(3):335–62.
39. Worling JR, Langstrom N. Assessment of criminal recidivism risk with adolescents who have offended sexually: a review. Trauma Violence Abuse 2003;4(4):341–62.
40. Christiansen AK, Vincent JP. Characterization and prediction of sexual and nonsexual recidivism among adjudicated juvenile sex offenders. Behav Sci Law 2013;31(4):506–29.
41. Pullman L, Seto MC. Assessment and treatment of adolescent sexual offenders: implications of recent research on generalist versus specialist explanations. Child Abuse Negl 2012;36(3):203–9.

42. Allnutt SH, Bradford JM, Greenberg DM, et al. Co-morbidity of alcoholism and the paraphilias. J Forensic Sci 1996;41(2):234–9.
43. DelBello MP, Soutullo CA, Zimmerman ME, et al. Traumatic brain injury in individuals convicted of sexual offenses with and without bipolar disorder. Psychiatry Res 1999;89(3):281–6.
44. McElroy SL, Soutullo CA, Taylor P Jr, et al. Psychiatric features of 36 men convicted of sexual offenses. J Clin Psychiatry 1999;60(6):414–20 [quiz: 421–2].
45. Raymond NC, Coleman E, Ohlerking F, et al. Psychiatric comorbidity in pedophilic sex offenders. Am J Psychiatry 1999;156(5):786–8.
46. Dwyer RG, Letourneau EJ. Juveniles who sexually offend: recommending a treatment program and level of care. Child Adolesc Psychiatr Clin N Am 2011;20(3): 413–29.
47. Fagan J, Wexler S. Explanations of sexual assault among violent delinquents. J Adolesc Res 1988;3:363–85.
48. Kavoussi RJ, Kaplan M, Becker JV. Psychiatric diagnoses in adolescent sex offenders. J Am Acad Child Adolesc Psychiatry 1988;27(2):241–3.
49. Hare RD. Psychopathy as a risk factor for violence. Psychiatr Q 1999;70(3): 181–97.
50. Parks GA, Bard DE. Risk factors for adolescent sex offender recidivism: evaluation of predictive factors and comparison of three groups based upon victim type. Sex Abuse 2006;18(4):319–42.
51. Edens JF, Skeem JL, Cruise KR, et al. Assessment of "juvenile psychopathy" and its association with violence: a critical review. Behav Sci Law 2001;19(1):53–80.
52. Vincent GM, Odgers CL, McCormick AV, et al. The PCL: YV and recidivism in male and female juveniles: a follow-up into young adulthood. Int J Law Psychiatry 2008;31(3):287–96.
53. Fazel S, Doll H, Langstrom N. Mental disorders among adolescents in juvenile detention and correctional facilities: a systematic review and metaregression analysis of 25 surveys. J Am Acad Child Adolesc Psychiatry 2008;47(9):1010–9.
54. Fazel S, Danesh J. Serious mental disorder in 23000 prisoners: a systematic review of 62 surveys. Lancet 2002;359(9306):545–50.
55. McClelland GM, Elkington KS, Teplin LA, et al. Multiple substance use disorders in juvenile detainees. J Am Acad Child Adolesc Psychiatry 2004;43(10):1215–24.
56. Abram KM, Teplin LA, Charles DR, et al. Posttraumatic stress disorder and trauma in youth in juvenile detention. Arch Gen Psychiatry 2004;61(4):403–10.
57. Abram KM, Washburn JJ, Teplin LA, et al. Posttraumatic stress disorder and psychiatric comorbidity among detained youths. Psychiatr Serv 2007;58(10):1311–6.
58. Abram KM, Choe JY, Washburn JJ, et al. Suicidal ideation and behaviors among youths in juvenile detention. J Am Acad Child Adolesc Psychiatry 2008;47(3): 291–300.
59. Finkelhor D, Ormrod R, Chaffin M, editors. Juveniles who commit sex offenses against minors. Washington, DC: Office of Juvenile Justice and Delinquency Prevention; 2009. Juvenile Justice Bulletin. NCJ227763.
60. Roe-Sepowitz D, Krysik J. Examining the sexual offenses of female juveniles: the relevance of childhood maltreatment. Am J Orthopsychiatry 2008;78(4): 405–12.
61. Cortoni F, Hanson RK, Coache ME. The recidivism rates of female sexual offenders are low: a meta-analysis. Sex Abuse 2010;22(4):387–401.
62. van der Put CE. The prevalence of risk factors for general recidivism in female adolescent sexual offenders: a comparison of three subgroups. Child Abuse Negl 2013;37(9):691–7.

63. van der Put C, van Vugt ES, Stams GJ, et al. Psychosocial and developmental characteristics of female adolescents who have committed sexual offenses. Sex Abuse 2013;26(4):330–42.
64. Hanson RK, Helmus L, Thornton D. Predicting recidivism amongst sexual offenders: a multi-site study of static-2002. Law Hum Behav 2009;34(3): 198–211.
65. Hanson RK, Thornton D. Static 99: improving actuarial risk assessment for sex offenders. 1999;User Rep 1999–02.
66. Prentky R, Righthand S, editors. Juvenile sex offender assessment protocol (J-SOAP-II): Manual. Bridgewater (MA): Justice Research Institute; 2003.
67. Hempel I, Buck N, Cima M, et al. Review of risk assessment instruments for juvenile sex offenders: what is next? Int J Offender Ther Comp Criminol 2013;57(2): 208–28.
68. Aebi M, Plattner B, Steinhausen HC, et al. Predicting sexual and nonsexual recidivism in a consecutive sample of juveniles convicted of sexual offences. Sex Abuse 2011;23(4):456–73.
69. Worling JR, Curwen T, editors. Estimated risk of adolescent sexual offense recidivism (ERASOR). Toronto: Ontario Ministry of Community and Social Services; 2001. Version 2.0 ed.
70. Viljoen JL, Mordell S, Beneteau JL. Prediction of adolescent sexual reoffending: a meta-analysis of the J-SOAP-II, ERASOR, J-SORRAT-II, and static-99. Law Hum Behav 2012;36(5):423–38.
71. Caldwell MF, Ziemke MH, Vitacco MJ. An examination of the sex offender registration act as applied to juveniles: examining the ability to predict sexual recidivism. Psychol Publ Pol Law 2008;14:89–114.
72. Letourneau EJ, Bandyopadhyay D, Sinha D, et al. Effects of sex offender registration policies on juvenile justice decision making. Sex Abuse 2009;21(2): 149–65.
73. Worling JR, Litteljohn A, Bookalam D. 20-year prospective follow-up study of specialized treatment for adolescents who offended sexually. Behav Sci Law 2010;28(1):46–57.
74. Hunter J. The effective management of juvenile sex offenders in the community: case management protocols. Virginia Department of Juvenile Justice. 2002. Available at: http://www.csom.org/pubs/JuvProtocols.pdf. Accessed September 28, 2015.
75. Hanson RK, Gordon A, Harris AJ, et al. First report of the collaborative outcome data project on the effectiveness of psychological treatment for sex offenders. Sex Abuse 2002;14(2):169–94 [discussion: 195–7].
76. Kolko DJ, Noel C, Thomas G, et al. Cognitive-behavioral treatment for adolescents who sexually offend and their families: individual and family applications in a collaborative outpatient program. J Child Sex Abus 2004;13(3–4):157–92.
77. Henggeler SW, Letourneau EJ, Chapman JE, et al. Mediators of change for multisystemic therapy with juvenile sexual offenders. J Consult Clin Psychol 2009; 77(3):451–62.
78. Letourneau EJ, Henggeler SW, McCart MR, et al. Two-year follow-up of a randomized effectiveness trial evaluating MST for juveniles who sexually offend. J Fam Psychol 2013;27(6):978–85.
79. Lipsey MW, Howell JC, Kelly MR, et al, editors. Inproving the effectiveness of juvenile justice programs: a new perspective on evidence-based parctice. Washington, DC: Georgetown Public Policy Institute; 2010. Available at:http://cjjr.georgetown.edu/pdfs/ebp/ebppaper.pdf.

80. Thibaut F, De La Barra F, Gordon H, et al, WFSBP Task Force on Sexual Disorders. The world federation of societies of biological psychiatry (WFSBP) guidelines for the biological treatment of paraphilias. World J Biol Psychiatry 2010;11(4): 604–55.
81. Bradford JM. The paraphilias, obsessive compulsive spectrum disorder, and the treatment of sexually deviant behaviour. Psychiatr Q 1999;70(3):209–19.
82. Bradford JM. The neurobiology, neuropharmacology, and pharmacological treatment of the paraphilias and compulsive sexual behaviour. Can J Psychiatry 2001; 46(1):26–34.
83. Mick TM, Hollander E. Impulsive-compulsive sexual behavior. CNS Spectr 2006; 11(12):944–55.
84. Aguirre B. Fluoxetine and compulsive sexual behavior. J Am Acad Child Adolesc Psychiatry 1999;38(8):943.
85. Galli VB, Raute NJ, McConville BJ, et al. An adolescent male with multiple paraphilias successfully treated with fluoxetine. J Child Adolesc Psychopharmacol 1998;8(3):195–7.
86. Ryan EP. Biological and pharmacological treatment. In: Ryan EP, Murrie DC, Hunter JA, editors. Juvenile sex offenders. New York: Oxford University Press; 2012. p. 193–238.

Juvenile Firesetting

Brittany Peters, MD, Bradley Freeman, MD*

KEYWORDS

• Firesetting • Delinquency • Arson • Conduct disorder • Juvenile

KEY POINTS

- There is a broad spectrum of psychological motivation behind juvenile firesetting behavior.
- Interventions with cognitive behavioral techniques and community resources have been helpful for these youth, whereas satiation has been counterproductive.
- Juvenile firesetting accounts for significant loss of life and property damage every year in the United States.
- Forensic assessment of firesetting youth involved with the juvenile justice system can help guide courts toward effective adjudication.

INTRODUCTION

Children and youth have an almost universal fascination with fire. From campfires, to fireplaces lit during the winter months, to fireworks on the fourth of July, almost nothing captures the attention of youth like fire. However, juveniles sometimes engage in dangerous behaviors associated with fire. These behaviors lead to significant morbidity and mortality in the United States in addition to hundreds of millions of dollars in property damage. Although arson, the criminal act of intentionally and maliciously setting fire to property, comprises one form of juvenile firesetting, juveniles may also set fire for other reasons and the consequences can be equally detrimental.

DEVELOPMENT OF FIRESETTING

Human beings are inherently interested in fire. Despite fire being potentially dangerous and destructive, evolutionary anthropologists such as Daniel Fessler[1] postulate that humans have developed an evolutionary advantage by being interested in fire and having the desire to control it. Fire can be used in cooking, forging hunting materials,

Disclosures: The authors have nothing to disclose.
Department of Psychiatry, Vanderbilt University School of Medicine, 1601 23rd Avenue South, Suite 3023, Nashville, TN 37212, USA
* Corresponding author.
E-mail address: bradley.w.freeman@vanderbilt.edu

Child Adolesc Psychiatric Clin N Am 25 (2016) 99–106
http://dx.doi.org/10.1016/j.chc.2015.08.009 **childpsych.theclinics.com**
1056-4993/16/$ – see front matter

and in combating enemies, and the ability to control smoke and fire has obvious safety implications.[1] Some level of fire interest is developmentally appropriate, and most children develop some curiosity about fire around the age of 3 years. The level of interest and risk associated with fire varies between individuals. Juvenile involvement with fire ranges from curiosity about fire and controlled, supervised fire starting to intentional firesetting and arson. The Federal Emergency Management Association has developed an extensive document describing assessment of children's interest in fire and determining children's risk categories based on assessment.[2] Such standardized assessments can be helpful in determining which children may benefit from further intervention when the level of potential risk is unclear.

SAFETY AND STATISTICS

The National Fire Protection Association (NFPA) reported that, between 2007 and 2011, 282,600 intentional fires were reported to US fire departments each year, with annual losses of 420 deaths, 1360 injuries, and $1.3 billion dollars in damaged property. Forty percent of individuals arrested for these events were less than 18 years of age.[3] In addition, the NFPA reports that during this time period 49,300 fires secondary to children playing with fire were reported to US fire departments, resulting in 80 deaths, 860 injuries, and an additional $230 million dollars in property damage.[4]

For children involved in firesetting behaviors, parents should be informed and encouraged to maintain a safe environment in the home as well as to provide increased supervision of their children. Depending on the intensity of the thoughts and behaviors, the family may need to inform the school, neighbors, and other adults who are in a position of providing supervision for the youth. Notably, fireplay has been noted to be the major cause of death among children in residential fires. The study also concluded that smoke alarms seemed to offer no protection from death or injury in fires caused by fireplay.[5] This evidence supports the need for close supervision and controlling access to fire starting or incendiary materials in the environment.

RISK FACTORS FOR JUVENILE FIRESETTING

Researchers have attempted to characterize juvenile firesetters based on demographic, psychological, and psychiatric data. However, there is little consensus regarding specific risk factors or characteristics common to all juvenile firesetters. Although there is a significant body of literature examining potential risk factors for firesetting behavior in juveniles, the factors explored in each study are widely variable. The evidence suggests that the cause for firesetting in juveniles is multifactorial and likely a complex interplay between environmental, psychological, and biological mechanisms. The most commonly explored risk factors are discussed in further detail later.

The concept of fire interest has consistently been associated with firesetting behavior in multiple studies and has been identified as a risk factor for recidivism.[6–9] In a study of 343 psychiatric patients, firesetters were distinguished from nonfiresetters by the intensity of their curiosity about fire.[10] Similarly, early experiences with fire, early exposure to firesetting, and previous intentional firesetting behaviors are associated with juvenile firesetting behavior.[10,11]

Being male is frequently reported as a risk factor for firesetting,[11–13] consistent with findings in the adult population, in which a study of 43,000 adults showed a 1.7% lifetime prevalence rate of firesetting in men and 0.4% in women.[13] Notably, female firesetters are more likely than male firesetters to have severe antisocial behaviors and issues with substance use.[14]

Substance use, specifically alcohol and cannabis, is another common risk factor identified in firesetting. One large study of 3965 students in grades 7 to 12 showed that binge drinking and frequent cannabis use are associated with firesetting behavior, and those individuals who use additional illicit substances are more likely to be high-frequency firesetters.[11]

Researchers have also evaluated the role of maltreatment in firesetting behavior. A study of 205 children aged 4 to 17 years reported that 48% of these children had experienced maltreatment and, compared with a nonmaltreated group, the children with history of maltreatment were more likely to have a history of firesetting and have more access to ignition sources.[15] This finding is consistent with reports that children with emotional and physical abuse are more likely to have a history of firesetting than nonabused children. In addition to physical and emotional abuse, experiencing peer rejection[16] and witnessing marital violence have shown strong correlations with firesetting behavior.[14]

The adult literature has suggested an association between psychiatric illness and firesetting behavior, particularly with affective disorders and substance use disorders.[17,18] For the child and adolescent population, the association between a specific psychiatric illnesses and firesetting is unclear. However, children with firesetting behaviors are more likely than other juvenile offenders to have received mental health treatment and to have had suicidal thoughts in the past.[19] Conduct disorder and attention-deficit/hyperactivity disorder (ADHD) have been associated with juvenile firesetting in some studies.[14,20] In addition, although it has long been suggested that firesetting, enuresis, and cruelty to animals exist as a triad in juvenile firesetters, this relationship has not held up under study.[21,22]

RECIDIVISM

Risk factors for recidivism, or relapse of criminal behavior, are important to consider given the implications for identifying high-risk individuals and developing appropriate therapeutic interventions. A study of 192 firesetters referred to an arson prevention program revealed that a parent report measure of fire interest was a predictor for severity of firesetting as well as recidivism.[23] Similarly, Kolko and colleagues[8] reported that curiosity of fire and covert antisocial behavior were associated with repeat firesetting offenses in a sample of 95 firesetters evaluated using a structured interview (**Table 1**).

Table 1
Risk factors and interventions for firesetting in juveniles

Factor	Intervention
Interest in/curiosity about fire	Parental supervision, psychoeducation, and possibly psychotherapy
Male gender	None
Substance use (especially alcohol and cannabis)	Treatment of substance use
History of maltreatment	Provide a safe and validating environment for the youth; psychotherapy
Psychiatric illness (especially conduct disorder and ADHD)	Treatment of the comorbid condition
Covert antisocial behavior	Multitier interventions such as multisystemic therapy

Consideration of the risk factors discussed earlier is important when evaluating a child because they may help to guide the clinician in determining what level of risk a particular child has with relationship to problematic firesetting behavior. In addition, notation of these risk factors can be helpful in determining what to include in an assessment of a child with potentially problematic firesetting behavior. For example, asking questions about the child's interest in fire and whether the child has been maltreated is more likely to be relevant than asking about nighttime enuresis.

TREATMENT

Investigators have evaluated the efficacy of a variety of interventions with regard to juvenile firesetting. In general, interventions have included educational programs and interventions based in cognitive behavior therapy (CBT). Many of these studies involve children referred for intervention from the juvenile justice system. It seems that another likely target population for intervention is children treated in burn centers as victims from fires they set themselves. Although most burn care facilities treating pediatric patients agree that having a tool to educate patients and families on the consequences of firesetting would be helpful, in a survey conducted by Ahrns-Klas and colleagues[24] only 38% of centers had such a program internally available, whereas another 38% of programs refer out because of lack of funds and staffing.

Cognitive Behavior Therapy–Based Intervention Programs

CBT is designed to assist individuals with connecting thoughts, feelings, and behaviors, and then to use this knowledge to adjust maladaptive thoughts and behaviors.[25] Because firesetting is a maladaptive behavior, CBT is a reasonable intervention to consider for behavior modification.

In the early 1980s, Bumpass and colleagues[26,27] studied a technique designed to interrupt firesetting. The technique attempted to help the child connect events, feelings, and behaviors around firesetting. This intervention was conducted by the investigators and, in a later study, conducted by firemen trained by the initial investigators. The investigators reported minimal repeat firesetting events (2 events in 29 patients) and increased improvement in outcomes and cost-efficiency compared with previously enacted community programs in the interventions conducted by firefighters.

CBT was compared with fire safety education or home visit with a firefighter in another study of 38 juvenile firesetters. CBT and fire safety education were reported to be superior to home visits with a firefighter with regard to the following outcomes: frequency of firesetting, playing with matches, severity of individualized problems with fire, involvement in fire-related acts, and "other deviant fire activities."[28] CBT is generally regarded as an acceptable and efficacious treatment to prevent future episodes of firesetting, although, as is the case in many of the described interventions, study numbers have been small and outcome measures are not uniform.

Pharmacotherapy

There are no medications indicated for the treatment of firesetting behaviors; however, this does not indicate that a medication trial is not warranted. Providers should consider firesetting behavior as a component of another psychiatric disorder until proved otherwise. Diagnoses to consider include the disruptive behaviors as well as mood, anxious, and psychotic disorders. Substance use is also over-represented in the adolescent population of firesetters. Identifying and treating a comorbid psychiatric condition may alleviate the firesetting behaviors.

Community Agency–Based Interventions

A variety of community-based interventions have been described in the literature. The programs described vary in relation to agencies involved, types of information disseminated, and outcomes measured. A large, prospective study was conducted to examine an intervention provided by a local fire district and regional burn center in Colorado. The program described took place over 2 half-days and included working with firemen and simulating response to a fire as well as touring a burn unit. Two-hundred and twenty juvenile firesetters participated in this program. Although all participants showed gains in general fire safety knowledge and knowledge of burn injuries, no changes within the home related to fire safety were made until parents were included in the intervention. Investigators reported that only 1 participant was referred back to the juvenile justice system for firesetting, but acknowledged that they did not have other active measurements of follow-up for recidivism.[29]

Another large study of 235 firesetting juveniles referred by the juvenile justice system compared the effects of education provided by the regional burn center with no education. The educational intervention consisted of teaching the juveniles the impact of firesetting behavior from a medical, financial, legal, and societal perspective. Study participants were tracked by the juvenile justice system and the fire department. Children who received the educational intervention had a significantly diminished recidivism rate (1 out of 32 vs 32 out of 102; odds ratio, 0.02; and $P<.001$) compared with children without intervention.[30]

Satiation

The process of satiation, or repeatedly lighting fire in a controlled setting to extinguish the desire to light fires, has been studied as a possible treatment of problematic firesetting and was once thought to be a useful intervention. However, studies have shown that satiation makes the child feel more competent around fire and is more likely to increase the behavior (**Table 2**).[31]

Clinician Resources

In addition to its comprehensive publication on juvenile firesetting intervention, the US Fire Administration and Federal Emergency Management Agency have produced fire safety education materials for a variety of audiences available on their Web site (www.usfa.fema.gov). Further fire safety education materials can be found on the Web site for state fire marshals (www.firemarshals.org). Several states have online resources available for families to use. Local fire departments are also often available to educate their communities about fire safety.

Table 2
Studied treatments for firesetting and their outcomes

Treatment	Focus	Outcome
CBT	Focusing on inciting events, thoughts, feelings, and firesetting behaviors	Positive
Pharmacotherapy	Comorbid conditions	Presumed positive
Fire and burn education	Psychoeducation about fire safety for the youth and family	Positive when a parent to the youth is also involved
Satiation	Eliminating the preoccupation of fire through overexposure	Negative

FORENSIC ASPECTS

Research concerning forensic aspects of fire setting behavior is sparse and scattered across the mental health, legal, and public safety literature. Various terms for firesetting behavior exist in the literature. These terms include fire interest, fireplay, fire involvement, firesetting, pathologic firesetting, arson, and pyromania. Each term conceptualizes the motivation and behavior toward fire differently. Some investigators offer a distinction between persons having fire interest and those who have fire involvement. Fire involvement suggests that the person has more than a preoccupation with fire and engages in fire-related behavior, which could be defined as firesetting or fireplay. Pathologic firesetting is caused by a psychological drive and is not necessarily the same as arson. Arson is broadly defined as an intentional criminal behavior in which an individual uses fire to inflict damage. With the publication of the Diagnostic and Statistical Manual of Mental Disorders, Fifth Edition , the diagnosis of pyromania has become obsolete because firesetting behaviors were thought to be better encapsulated within other diagnoses, such as conduct disorder.[32]

Youth may become involved in the juvenile justice system because of firesetting behaviors. Understanding the thought process behind the behavior helps to provide effective interventions. For instance, a motivation to harm requires different intervention than simple fireplay in which there is no intention for harm. When damage has resulted from firesetting, the line between criminal and noncriminal motivation can be difficult to distinguish. Forensic experts help educate the court and legal system about the behaviors as well as provide thoughtful assessments of youth to guide the courts in the decision-making process.[33]

DISCUSSION

Intervening with juveniles who have engaged in firesetting or who report a preoccupation with fire can be lifesaving. Psychotherapeutic and community interventions are available for these youth. With regard to therapy, CBT-based interventions have been helpful, whereas fire satiation has been shown to be counterproductive. Concerning community-based treatments, positive effects were appreciated when at least 1 of the child's parents was also engaged in the intervention. Community programs are occasionally provided through the public school system to students early in their education. Youth who become involved in the juvenile justice system may benefit from an expert evaluation. Forensic experts can attempt to describe the child's motivation and offer appropriate intervention recommendations that may help steer the court away from a punitive perspective and focus on treatment/rehabilitation.

The research regarding firesetting in youth is growing. Additional investigation into the various motivations for firesetting and its relation to other psychiatric disorders, including personality disorders, would be welcomed. Providers should conduct fire safety discussions with the family, especially if their youth is identified as a firesetter or has a preoccupation with fire. The discussion should focus on the need to limit access to incendiary devices/materials, the need for increased supervision, and providing resources to the family. One helpful resource is the family's local fire department. Fire departments typically provide community education, handouts, and home inspections for fire safety.

REFERENCES

1. Fessler D. A burning desire: steps toward an evolutionary psychology of fire learning. J Cognit Cult 2006;6:431–51.

2. Gaynor J. Juvenile firesetter intervention handbook. Emmitsburg (MD): Administration USF; 2002.
3. Campbell R. Intentional fires. Quincy (MA): Association NFP; 2014.
4. Campbell R. Playing with fire. Quincy (MA): Association NFP; 2014.
5. Istre GR, McCoy M, Carlin DK, et al. Residential fire related deaths and injuries among children: fireplay, smoke alarms, and prevention. Inj Prev 2002;8:128–32.
6. Del Bove G, Caprara GV, Pastorelli C, et al. Juvenile firesetting in Italy: relationship to aggression, psychopathology, personality, self-efficacy, and school functioning. Eur Child Adolesc Psychiatry 2008;17:235–44.
7. Kolko DJ, Day BT, Bridge JA, et al. Two-year prediction of children's firesetting in clinically referred and nonreferred samples. J Child Psychol Psychiatry 2001;42:371–80.
8. Kolko DJ, Kazdin AE. Children's descriptions of their firesetting incidents: characteristics and relationship to recidivism. J Am Acad Child Adolesc Psychiatry 1994;33:114–22.
9. Gannon TA, Ciardha CO, Barnoux MF, et al. Male imprisoned firesetters have different characteristics than other imprisoned offenders and require specialist treatment. Psychiatry 2013;76:349–64.
10. Kolko DJ, Kazdin AE. Assessment of dimensions of childhood firesetting among patients and nonpatients: the firesetting risk interview. J Abnorm Child Psychol 1989;17:157–76.
11. MacKay S, Paglia-Boak A, Henderson J, et al. Epidemiology of firesetting in adolescents: mental health and substance use correlates. J Child Psychol Psychiatry 2009;50:1282–90.
12. Lambie I, Ioane J, Randell I, et al. Offending behaviours of child and adolescent firesetters over a 10-year follow-up. J Child Psychol Psychiatry 2013;54:1295–307.
13. Hoertel N, Le Strat Y, Schuster JP, et al. Gender differences in firesetting: results from the National Epidemiologic Survey on Alcohol and Related Conditions (NESARC). Psychiatry Res 2011;190:352–8.
14. Becker KD, Stuewig J, Herrera VM, et al. A study of firesetting and animal cruelty in children: family influences and adolescent outcomes. J Am Acad Child Adolesc Psychiatry 2004;43:905–12.
15. Root C, Mackay S, Henderson J, et al. The link between maltreatment and juvenile firesetting: correlates and underlying mechanisms. Child Abuse Negl 2008;32:161–76.
16. Chen YH, Arria AM, Anthony JC. Firesetting in adolescence and being aggressive, shy, and rejected by peers: new epidemiologic evidence from a national sample survey. J Am Acad Psychiatry Law 2003;31:44–52.
17. Labree W, Nijman H, van Marle H, et al. Backgrounds and characteristics of arsonists. Int J Law Psychiatry 2010;33:149–53.
18. Ducat L, Ogloff JR, McEwan T. Mental illness and psychiatric treatment amongst firesetters, other offenders and the general community. Aust N Z J Psychiatry 2013;47:945–53.
19. Rasanen P, Hirvenoja R, Hakko H, et al. A portrait of the juvenile arsonist. Forensic Sci Int 1995;73:41–7.
20. Kolko DJ. Handbook on firesetting in children and youth. San Diego (CA): Academic Press; 2002.
21. Showers J, Pickrell E. Child firesetters: a study of three populations. Hosp Community Psychiatry 1987;38:495–501.

22. Slavkin ML. Enuresis, firesetting, and cruelty to animals: does the ego triad show predictive validity? Adolescence 2001;36:461–6.
23. MacKay S, Henderson J, Del Bove G, et al. Fire interest and antisociality as risk factors in the severity and persistence of juvenile firesetting. J Am Acad Child Adolesc Psychiatry 2006;45:1077–84.
24. Ahrns-Klas KS, Wahl WL, Hemmila MR, et al. Do burn centers provide juvenile firesetter intervention? J Burn Care Res 2012;33:272–8.
25. Beck JS. Cognitive behavior therapy: basics and beyond. 2nd edition. New York: The Guilford Press; 2011.
26. Bumpass ER, Brix RJ, Preston D. A community-based program for juvenile firesetters. Hosp Community Psychiatry 1985;36:529–33.
27. Bumpass ER, Fagelman FD, Brix RJ. Intervention with children who set fires. Am J Psychother 1983;37:328–45.
28. Kolko DJ. Efficacy of cognitive-behavioral treatment and fire safety education for children who set fires: initial and follow-up outcomes. J Child Psychol Psychiatry 2001;42:359–69.
29. Carroll W, Austgen W, Hansbrough J, et al. The development of a program for juvenile fire offenders. J Burn Care Rehabil 1986;7:253–6.
30. Franklin GA, Pucci PS, Arbabi S, et al. Decreased juvenile arson and firesetting recidivism after implementation of a multidisciplinary prevention program. J Trauma 2002;53:260–4 [discussion: 264–6].
31. Sharp DBS, Cole E, Cole R. Evidence-based multidisciplinary strategies for working with children who set fires. J Am Psychiatr Nurses Assoc 2005;11:329–37.
32. American Psychiatric Association: recent updates to proposed revisions for DSM-5 | APA DSM-5. 2015. Available at: http://www.dsm5.org/Pages/RecentUpdates.aspx. Accessed June 1, 2015.
33. Burton PR, McNiel DE, Binder RL. Firesetting, arson, pyromania, and the forensic mental health expert. J Am Acad Psychiatry Law 2012;40:355–65.

Understanding and Responding to the Needs of Commercially Sexually Exploited Youth

Recommendations for the Mental Health Provider

Roya Ijadi-Maghsoodi, MD[a,b,*], Mekeila Cook, PhD[c],
Elizabeth S. Barnert, MD, MPH, MS[d],
Shushanik Gaboian, MSW[e], Eraka Bath, MD[f]

KEYWORDS

- Commercially sexually exploited children
- Commercial sexual exploitation of children • Sex trafficking • Human trafficking
- Exploitation

KEY POINTS

- Mental health providers may encounter commercially sexually exploited youth in various health care settings, emergency rooms, the juvenile justice system, and child welfare system.

Continued

Dr R. Ijadi-Maghsoodi is supported by the VA Office of Academic Affiliations through the VA Advanced Fellowship in Women's Health. Dr E. Bath receives funding from the NIMH (2P20 MD000182) and the Los Angeles County Department of Probation. Dr R. Ijadi-Maghsoodi, Dr E.S. Barnert, Dr M. Cook, and Ms S. Gaboian have nothing to disclose. The views expressed in this article are those of the authors and do not necessarily reflect the position or policy of the US Department of Veterans Affairs or the United States Government.
[a] VA HSR&D Center for the Study of Healthcare Innovation, Implementation & Policy, VA Greater Los Angeles Healthcare System, 11301 Wilshire Boulevard, Building 500, Room 1601, Office of Healthcare, Transformation and Innovation, Mail Code 10–C, Los Angeles, CA 90073, USA; [b] Department of Medicine, David Geffen School of Medicine, University of California Los Angeles, Los Angeles, CA 90095, USA; [c] Integrated Substance Abuse Programs, Department of Psychiatry and Biobehavioral Sciences, Semel Institute for Neuroscience and Human Behavior, University of California, Los Angeles, 11075 Santa Monica Boulevard, Suite 100, Los Angeles, CA 90025, USA; [d] Department of Pediatrics, David Geffen School of Medicine, University of California Los Angeles, Los Angeles, CA 90095, USA; [e] Department of Neuroscience and Human Behavior, University of California Los Angeles, Los Angeles, CA 90095, USA; [f] Child Forensic Services, Department of Psychiatry and Biobehavioral Sciences, Semel Institute for Neuroscience and Human Behavior, University of California Los Angeles, 300 Medical Plaza, Room 1243, Los Angeles, CA 90095, USA
* Corresponding author.
E-mail address: rijadimaghsoodi@mednet.ucla.edu

Child Adolesc Psychiatric Clin N Am 25 (2016) 107–122
http://dx.doi.org/10.1016/j.chc.2015.08.007
1056-4993/16/$ – see front matter Published by Elsevier Inc.
childpsych.theclinics.com

Continued

- Commercially sexually exploited youth are at risk for a variety of health and mental health issues, including posttraumatic stress disorder, depression, substance abuse, anxiety, and suicidality.
- Psychosocial risk factors contributing to identifying commercially sexually exploited youth include histories of abuse/neglect, foster care placement, running away, and homelessness.
- A trauma-informed, multidisciplinary approach incorporating evidenced-based practice and comprehensive case coordination is necessary to effectively address the needs of commercially sexually exploited youth.
- Techniques providers should use with these youth include establishing a safe environment by interviewing youth alone, providing an empathetic, nonjudgmental approach, and avoiding discussions that could revictimize youth.

INTRODUCTION

Commercial sexual exploitation of children (CSEC) is a critical human rights and public health issue that child psychiatrists and other mental health providers can play an important role in addressing. Although commercially sexually exploited youth often go unidentified by health providers, these youth may have frequent contact with health care, juvenile delinquency, and foster care systems, and therefore, likely interact with mental health providers who work in these settings. Although the data on commercially sexually exploited youth are limited, studies show that these youth are at high risk for medical and psychiatric problems and have challenging psychosocial histories, including having experienced childhood abuse, homelessness, and foster care placement.[1–4] The exact numbers of commercially sexually exploited youth are unknown given the clandestine nature of the exploitation and underreporting. Experts suggest that the number of sexually exploited children in the United States may be growing.[1] Understanding the risk factors for commercial sexual exploitation, the health and mental health implications, and treatment options can help improve detection and care for this underserved population.

DEFINING COMMERCIAL SEXUAL EXPLOITATION OF CHILDREN

To better understand CSEC, it is helpful to review the definition of human trafficking in its various forms, both internationally and in the United States. Trafficking in persons (also referred to as human trafficking) is defined by the United Nations Palermo Protocol as "the recruitment, transportation, transfer, harbouring or receipt of persons, by means of threat or use of force or other forms of coercion, of abduction, of fraud, of deception, or the abuse of power or of a position of vulnerability or of the giving or receiving of payments or benefits to achieve the consent of a person having control over another person for the purpose of exploitation."[5] Related to this, exploitation includes but is not limited to sexual exploitation, prostitution, forced labor, slavery, and servitude or the removal of organs.[5] Under the Palermo protocol, the trafficking of a child refers to all youth less than 18 years old.

In the United States, the Trafficking Victims Protection Act (TVPA) of 2000 provided a similar definition for victims of trafficking. The TVPA defined sex trafficking as the "recruitment, harboring, transportation, provision, or obtaining of a person for the purpose of a commercial sex act."[6] The TVPA defined severe trafficking as sex trafficking through the use of force, fraud, or coercion, or if the victim is less than 18 years of age.[6]

This definition means that a sex-trafficked child (less than 18 years old) is considered a victim of severe trafficking under the federal law due to age, without the requirement of the trafficker using force, fraud, or coercion. Under the law, physical transportation of a victim need not occur for a crime to be considered trafficking.

The term "commercial sexual exploitation of children" is defined by the Office of Juvenile Justice and Delinquency Prevention (OJJDP) as "crimes of a sexual nature committed against juvenile victims for financial or other economic reasons."[7] Sexual exploitation includes prostitution, pornography, sex tourism, mail order bride, adolescent marriage (generally to older men), performance in sexual venues such as strip clubs, survival sex, private parties, massage parlors, gang-based prostitution, and Internet-based exploitation.[7–9] Although not included in the legal definition by OJJDP, many experts also include youth who engage in sex for desirable items, perceived excitement, or social status, as well as those who in engage in "survival sex" (eg, engaging in sex acts in exchange for money, food, shelter, or other basic necessities) under the rubric of CSEC.[7,10] The terminology CSEC reflects an important shift in the paradigm of how these youth are perceived by the general public, by law enforcement, and by lawmakers, as well as by the legislative trends of decriminalization and diversion of trafficked victims.

The Trafficking Victims Protection Act of 2000 and "Safe Harbor" Protections for Commercially Sexually Exploited Youth

The TVPA of 2000, the first comprehensive federal human trafficking bill, addressed the prevention of human trafficking, provided a definition for victims of trafficking, authorized protections and assistance for victims, and increased penalties for traffickers.[6]

Although the passage of the TVPA signified a reorientation of federal policy toward trafficking victims, laws in all 50 states still classified commercially sexually exploited youth as criminals who could be incarcerated for prostitution.[7,11] In response, several states enacted "Safe Harbor" laws designed to reclassify youth as victims and ensure access to services and legal protections. These laws function to decriminalize juvenile prostitution such that victims can no longer be convicted for their exploitation or establish diversion pathways that redirect victims from the justice system into child welfare or specialized services.[11] New York enacted the Safe Harbor law in 2008.[12] By 2014, 22 states had enacted antitrafficking legislation that included various Safe Harbor protections.[13] In addition, Congress is again considering legislation that would incentivize all states to adopt Safe Harbor laws.[13]

Risk Factors Contributing to Vulnerability to Commercial Sexual Exploitation of Children

When addressing the legal protections and services these youth need, it is helpful to conceptualize CSEC within an ecological framework (**Fig. 1**). The ecological perspective acknowledges the distinct connection between the youth and the physical and sociocultural environment in which the youth interacts. The contact between and the interdependence of these risk outcomes are inextricably tied to interactions between each level: individual risk factors, family factors/dynamics, neighborhood/community living conditions, institutions and systems of care, social and legal policies.[14] Applying these principles is useful to understanding commercially sexually exploited youth as well as guiding treatment and community interventions. Although the factors that place youth at increased risk for commercial sexual exploitation are numerous, there are several psychosocial risks factors that have been frequently documented in youth who are commercially sexually exploited. These include,

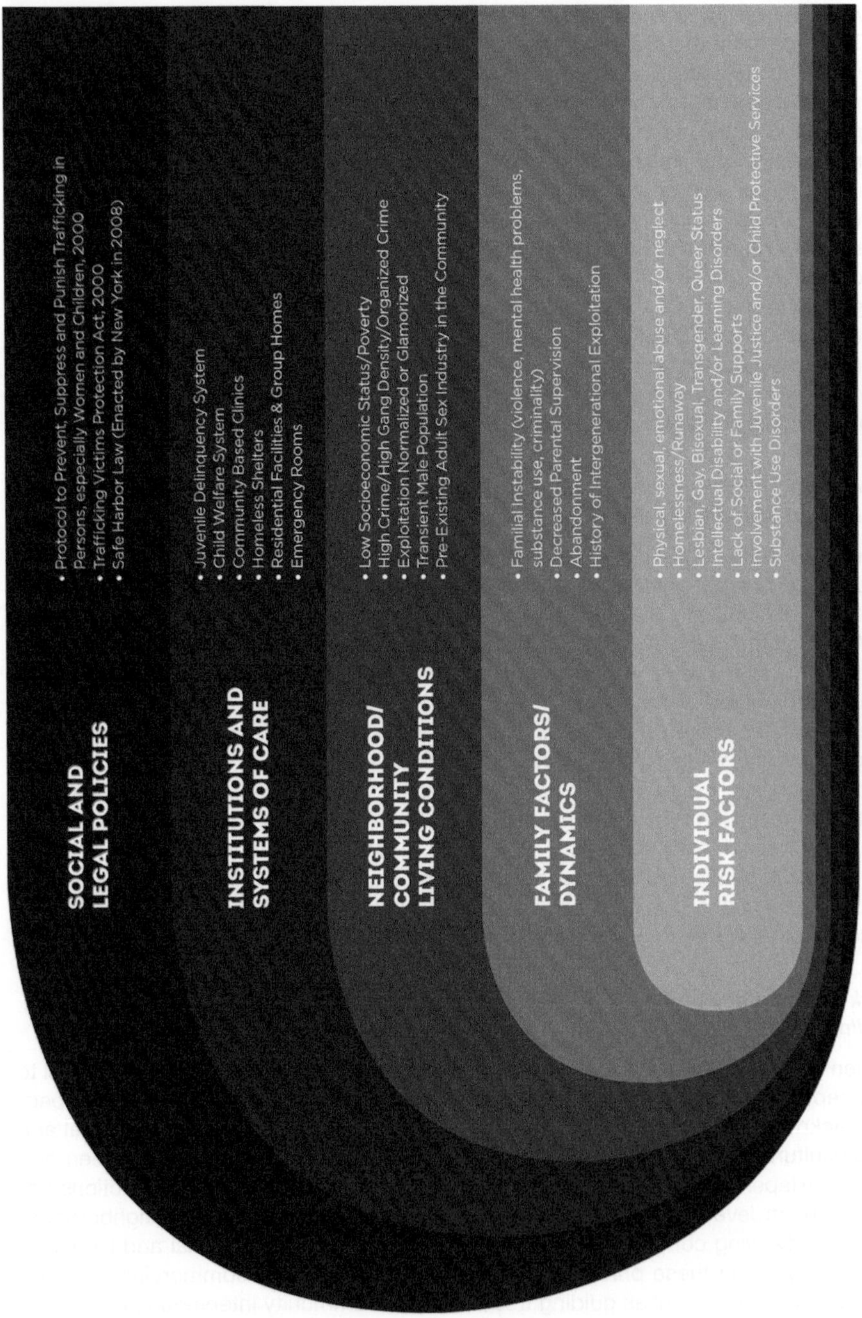
SOCIAL AND
LEGAL POLICIES
• Protocol to Prevent, Suppress and Punish Trafficking in Persons, especially Women and Children, 2000
• Trafficking Victims Protection Act, 2000
• Safe Harbor Law (Enacted by New York in 2008)
INSTITUTIONS AND
SYSTEMS OF CARE
• Juvenile Delinquency System
• Child Welfare System
• Community Based Clinics
• Homeless Shelters
• Residential Facilities & Group Homes
• Emergency Rooms
NEIGHBORHOOD/
COMMUNITY
LIVING CONDITIONS
• Low Socioeconomic Status/Poverty
• High Crime/High Gang Density/Organized Crime
• Exploitation Normalized or Glamorized
• Transient Male Population
• Pre-Existing Adult Sex Industry in the Community
FAMILY FACTORS/
DYNAMICS
• Familial Instability (violence, mental health problems, substance use, criminality)
• Decreased Parental Supervision
• Abandonment
• History of Intergenerational Exploitation
INDIVIDUAL
RISK FACTORS
• Physical, sexual, emotional abuse and/or neglect
• Homelessness/Runaway
• Lesbian, Gay, Bisexual, Transgender, Queer Status
• Intellectual Disability and/or Learning Disorders
• Lack of Social or Family Supports
• Involvement with Juvenile Justice and/or Child Protective Services
• Substance Use Disorders

Fig. 1. Ecological Framework for Contextualizing and Conceptualizing Commercial Sexual Exploitation of Children.

but are not limited to, childhood abuse, neglect, foster care placement, and homelessness.[1,15–18]

It is important for mental health clinicians to be aware of sexually exploited youth within the child welfare and juvenile justice system. Foster youth are at high risk for becoming exploited because they may have underlying histories of abuse that make them more vulnerable, and they may be in settings where they are at greater risk of victimization (eg, group homes, foster homes) and more accessible to potential traffickers or peers involved in trafficking.[1] Commercially sexually exploited youth also frequently present in the juvenile delinquency system. Although there has been a shift in many jurisdictions toward diverting commercially sexually exploited youth out of the juvenile delinquency system, youth are often first identified within the delinquency system after getting arrested for trafficking or non-trafficking-related offenses. Practitioners who work in the child welfare or juvenile justice settings are likely aware of the bidirectional flow of youth (commercially sexually exploited or otherwise) between these settings; this highlights an important point of contact for early detection by practitioners in both the child welfare and the juvenile justice settings.

Mental health providers should also be aware of the association between childhood abuse and being trafficked. One study reported the prevalence of emotional, physical, and sexual abuse in childhood among sexually exploited youth to be between 32% and 93%.[19] Researchers have documented the association between experiencing childhood sexual abuse and CSEC.[1,19] Experiencing childhood emotional abuse is also significantly associated with being trafficked[19] and with younger ages of entry into the commercial sex industry.[17] Experts hypothesize that the psychologically damaging effects of childhood abuse may affect one's sense of self-efficacy and coping in dangerous, high-risk situations; this in turn may place one at increased susceptibility to sexual victimization and commercial sexual exploitation.[17,19]

Another significant risk factor for commercial sexual exploitation is being homeless, including being a runaway or "thrown away" youth.[20,21] Many homeless youth who have fled situations of abuse and neglect must develop means of financial support in often-dangerous environments. Homeless youth often lack trusted social connections and thus are especially vulnerable to the exploitative techniques used by traffickers.[1] Indeed, among youth who entered the sex industry, a history of running away in childhood is associated with youth entering the sex industry under the age of 18 compared with women who enter over the age of 18.[17] It is estimated that 70% of youth living on the street engage in commercial sex to meet basic needs.[1]

Although historically undetected by outreach organizations that may focus efforts on heterosexual women, LGBTQ (lesbian, gay, bisexual, transgender, and queer) youth are at risk for commercial sexual exploitation due to their high risk for social marginalization, vulnerability to victimization, and homelessness.[22] One study examining risk factors among homeless youth for initiation into the street economy (including sexual exploitation) found that male-to-female transgender youth were especially vulnerable to exploitation given the barriers of stigma and discrimination to obtaining jobs in the formal economy.[23]

RECRUITMENT AND ENTRAPMENT TECHNIQUES USED BY TRAFFICKERS

The psychosocial context and the aforementioned risk factors place these youth at heightened vulnerability to the tactics used to recruit and maintain youth in commercial sexual exploitation. These techniques are important for mental health clinicians to understand, because they have the potential to affect the therapeutic relationship, the assessment, and the treatment of trafficked youth.

Domestic Recruitment

In the United States, youth may enter into the commercial sex industry through 4 main routes: by peer networks, by recruitment by sex traffickers directly (in-person or online), by abduction, or by being sold by family members.[1,10,18]

Research on recruitment through peer networks shows that this experience is more common than often realized. A study of commercially sexually exploited youth from New York revealed that 46% of the female youths and 44% of the male youths in the sample reported initiation by friends.[18] This recruitment process may occur through "friends" who are actually surrogate recruiters for pimps, through peers who help directly introduce youth to prostitution, or through social networks, where prostitution is normalized and glamorized and youth may be pressured to join.[18,23] Youth may be recruited in foster care homes, group facilities, or while homeless.

Another described path into sex trafficking is through exploitation by sex traffickers, commonly referred to by commercially sexually exploited youth as "pimp," "boyfriend," "sugar daddy," or "daddy."[16,24] Youth report that pimps may be men or women, known acquaintances, a "boyfriend" with likely ulterior motives from the beginning, or strangers.[16,18] Many traffickers use social media sites, such as Facebook and Twitter, to recruit youth.

It is known that traffickers target vulnerable adolescent girls using a variety of sophisticated coercive techniques, often dubbed "grooming techniques." These grooming techniques include romancing young adolescent girls; building trust, such as helping take care of vulnerable adolescents or helping them out of difficult situations; glamorizing and normalizing prostitution, through the use of jokes and luring them via female friends; isolating youth from their loved ones and home; abducting youth; and coercing youth via drugs and by debt bondage.[15] Reports also describe recruitment within gangs and recruitment of youth with intellectual disabilities.[15] One study of trafficked youth described that younger pimps tend to use violence or threats against girls, while older, likely more experienced pimps were known to manipulate youth through "smooth talking," promises of romance, and emotional control.[16] In many cases, a vulnerable youth is enticed into a relationship with a "boyfriend" through gifts, dates, and attention. A "trauma bond" is then formed with the exploiter, in which the youth is willing to do what the exploiter asks, including sex acts with others, to preserve the relationship. Frequently, the relationship descends into intimidation and violence.[10]

Enmeshment techniques used by sex traffickers include blackmailing, shaming, financial control, isolation, and using children and pregnancy, including threatening abortion or adoption of one's child, to control victims. Trafficked youth also report intimidation and threats of injury or death and physical violence.[15] Believing that the relationship is consensual and special, many sexually exploited youth develop feelings of obligation to their trafficker, unaware that they are being exploited.[2,15,16]

International Recruitment

Human traffickers involved in international trafficking may use similar manipulative mechanisms as pimps to recruit victims, including the use of fraud or force. International studies reveal that women and children often enter trafficking through collusion by a parent or friend.[4,25] Youth may also be pressured by family members to find work abroad, may be seeking a better life or financial opportunity, or may attempt migrating to escape political or domestic violence at home or in their country of origin. Youth migrating as unaccompanied minors are inherently vulnerable to exploitation through the migration process or may become victims of commercial sexual exploitation on arriving at their destination through being forced to pay back debt to traffickers.[1] Internationally trafficked youth often fear reprisals against their families in their country of origin and fear contacting service agencies and law enforcement in the United States, which heightens their vulnerability. Thus, traffickers often exert a higher level of control over these victims. As a result, the exploitation of internationally trafficked youth can be less visible.[1,25]

THE PSYCHIATRIC INTERVIEW AND POTENTIAL CHALLENGES

Given the complex psychological factors involved in the recruitment, entrapment, and enmeshment of commercially sexually exploited youth, obtaining an accurate history and assessment of trafficked youth may be difficult. Sexually exploited youth may distrust the interviewer, may have a desire to protect the perpetrator, and may fear retribution from their exploiter.[25,26] They may not realize they are being exploited and can be hesitant or unable to describe their traumatic experiences.[2,25] Shame and stigma have been described as major barriers to victims seeking mental health services.[26]

Because of these factors, providers must interview the youth alone, keeping in mind that they may be accompanied to health visits by an exploiter. Providers need to discuss confidentiality with the adolescent in the beginning, including what information must be reported under mandatory reporting laws; these laws differ by state and locality.[10] Given the traumatic and coercive situations many of these youth have endured, allowing the youth to feel empowered and in control of the situation and avoiding discussions and actions that could potentially revictimize the youth or make them feel threatened are vital.[26]

It is also important for the provider to establish an environment of safety and trust. Developing a therapeutic alliance may take time and repeated visits. Providing an empathic, partnered, nonjudgmental approach as well as avoiding the use of medical or legal jargon is also helpful. In one qualitative study examining how outreach workers could best engage trafficked youth, youth specifically reported that they wanted outreach workers to use milder words expressed in the youth's own language to describe sexual exploitation, including terms such as "working" or engaging in "the game." In this study, the youth also described wanting outreach workers to listen and care.[24]

IDENTIFICATION OF COMMERCIALLY SEXUALLY EXPLOITED YOUTH

Although trafficked youth likely will not self-identify as victims of sexual exploitation, these youth present for medical treatment, including in emergency rooms, reproductive health clinics, and community health centers. Psychiatrists and mental health providers may be asked to consult on these youth in hospitals and after they present to emergency departments. As described earlier, mental health providers may also encounter sexually exploited youth in the child welfare and justice systems.

Many organizations and agencies have identified physical and psychological signs as well as psychosocial history indicators that suggest a youth may be trafficked (**Box 1**). For example, the exploiter may accompany the youth to the medical visit. The youth may appear to be controlled or submissive to this person and may give false or changing information.[27] Although not all youth will display these signs, and having these characteristics does not mean that a youth is being sexually exploited, understanding the indicators and risk factors associated with commercially sexually exploited youth may improve identification and guide further assessment. Increasing detection of trafficked youth among health and mental health providers is essential for improving care for this population. In one study of female adult and adolescent

Box 1
Psychiatric interview: potential associated signs, mental health symptoms, and red flags for detecting commercially sexually exploited youth

Appearance and behavior

Youth is accompanied by an individual that appears controlling or does not want the youth to be interviewed alone

Youth displays a withdrawn, frightened, or guarded affect

Youth gives vague or changing demographic information

Youth appears intoxicated or impaired by substance use

Youth has evidence of branding or tattoos (including facial tattoos, gang-related tattoos)

Youth has evidence of physical injury (scars, burns, lacerations, fractures, traumatic brain injury)

Youth appears to be in poor physical health (evidence of skin infections, poor dentition, malnourishment)

Youth is carrying large amounts of money or expensive items that appear beyond the youth's means

Social history

Youth has a history of homelessness (includes running away, being abandoned, or forced to leave home)

Youth has an older boyfriend and/or history of multiple sexual partners

Youth has a history of juvenile justice system involvement

Youth has a history of involvement with child welfare services (including living in a group home/foster care home)

Youth does not attend school or is frequently truant

Medical history

Youth has a history of pregnancy, abortion, ectopic pregnancies

Youth has a history of multiple sexually transmitted diseases, pelvic inflammatory disease

Youth has frequent emergency room visits (including for physical injuries, reproductive concerns, or sexually transmitted diseases)

Mental health symptoms

Youth has symptoms of depression

Youth is suicidal

Youth has symptoms of posttraumatic stress disorder, traumatic stress, and/or anxiety symptoms

Youth has symptoms of a substance use disorder

Youth has problems with anger

Youth has self-harming behaviors

Having these signs does not mean that a child is being commercially sexually exploited, and lack of these signs does not rule out that a child is being commercially sexually exploited.

Adapted from Greenbaum VJ. Commercial sexual exploitation and sex trafficking of children in the United States. Curr Probl Pediatr Adolesc Health Care 2014;44(9):245–69; with permission. *Data from* Refs.[2,4,18,27,39]

trafficking survivors, 28% of survivors came into contact with a medical provider without being detected as a victim of trafficking.[25]

MENTAL HEALTH IMPLICATIONS OF COMMERCIAL SEXUAL EXPLOITATION OF CHILDREN

High rates of childhood maltreatment, exposure to violence, threats of death, coercion, isolation, and poor living situations create an environment where commercially sexually exploited youth are at elevated risk for severe mental health issues. These diagnoses include posttraumatic stress disorder (PTSD), depression, substance abuse, anxiety, and suicidality.[2–4]

One study of sexually exploited youth engaged in care in Northern California revealed high levels of depression, anxiety, anger problems, and attachment problems. In addition, more than 30% of the youth engaged in moderate to severe self-harming behavior.[2] Seventy-seven percent of trafficked women and adolescents receiving posttrafficking care in Europe met criteria for probable PTSD.[3] Cognitive impairment may also be encountered among sexually exploited youth, which could be secondary to traumatic brain injury and physical violence, or associated with mental health symptoms. In one study, almost two-thirds of the trafficked women reported memory problems.[4]

Substance use may also present with mental health problems and may exacerbate both mental health and physical health issues of trafficked youth. Youth may be forced to use, carry, or sell substances by exploiters, or may use substances to cope. Interviews with sexually exploited youth in New York City revealed that drug use was common, with more than 50% of the sample reporting regular marijuana use as well as the use of cocaine and alcohol.[18]

PHYSICAL HEALTH IMPLICATIONS OF COMMERCIAL SEXUAL EXPLOITATION OF CHILDREN

Along with the adverse effects on mental health, CSEC has profound immediate and long-term detrimental effects on physical health with important implications for the psychiatrist (**Box 2**). Understanding these potential health needs may facilitate needed medical referrals and improve the overall quality of care for this high-risk, medically underserved group.

Commercially sexually exploited youth have high rates of violence-related injuries and unmet reproductive health needs.[10] A report on trafficked women and adolescents receiving services in Europe described that 76% of the women reported physical violence during trafficking, and 90% reported sexual violence.[4] Similarly, a cross-sectional study of female domestic sex trafficking victims found that 89% reported experiencing physical violence; 59% reported having a sexually transmitted infection, and 58% became pregnant while trafficked.[28]

High rates of injection drug use and unsafe sex make sexually exploited youth especially vulnerable to infectious diseases, such as HIV and hepatitis C.[10] In addition, despite the fact that more than three-quarters of sexually exploited youth report having seen a medical provider within the past 6 months, these youth also have higher rates of malnutrition, general infections, and untreated chronic medical conditions, such as asthma, diabetes, and sickle-cell anemia.[10,18] Psychiatrists can serve an important role in directing commercially sexually exploited youth to needed medical care and should also take into consideration the potential psychological trauma and needs that may result from the medical conditions experienced by these youth.

Box 2
Physical health implications of commercial sexual exploitation of children for the mental health provider

Violence-related injury

- Commercially sexually exploited youth may be in immediate physical danger. Providers can assess current safety as a priority.
- Commercially sexually exploited youth may have acute injuries (eg, lacerations, fractures, traumatic brain injury, anogenital trauma) requiring immediate medical care or may be suffering from physical or mental health sequelae from previous violent-related injuries.
- Providers can assess the need for referral for acute medical care and address psychological trauma related to previous violent injuries.

Reproductive health needs

- Most commercially sexually exploited youth practice unsafe sex at least some of the time. Providers can encourage youth to practice abstinence (if feasible) or safe sex practices.
- Rates of sexually transmitted infections, such as chlamydia, gonorrhea, HIV, and syphilis, are disproportionately high. Providers can administer testing or offer referrals for testing and treatment of sexually transmitted infections.
- Commercially sexually exploited youth have high rates of current pregnancy or abortions or have already had children (many of whom have been removed from their custody). Providers can offer pregnancy testing (or referral for testing) and explore psychological trauma related to pregnancies, parenthood, and/or abortions.

Infectious diseases

- Infections, such as endocarditis, tuberculosis, and untreated dental caries, may be more common in commercially sexually exploited youth.
- By building trust with youth and providing necessary medical referrals, providers can play an important role in connecting commercially sexually exploited youth to needed medical care.

Chronic medical conditions

- Commercially sexually exploited youth are more likely to have untreated chronic conditions, such as asthma, diabetes, and sickle-cell disease.
- Providers can help assess barriers to medical care and provide referrals to medical providers.

Substance use

- Underlying substance use strongly affects the physical health of commercially sexually exploited youth. It contributes to conditions such as malnutrition, infections, and unsafe sexual practices.
- By addressing substance use and abuse, providers can fulfill a critical role in improving the physical health of commercially sexually exploited youth.

Adapted from Greenbaum VJ. Commercial sexual exploitation and sex trafficking of children in the United States. Curr Probl Pediatr Adolesc Health Care 2014;44(9):245–69; with permission. *Data from* Refs.[18,28]

TREATMENT OPTIONS AND APPROACHES

Despite a growing interest among providers, policymakers, and researchers in understanding the needs and providing services to sexually exploited youth, evidence-based research studies and program evaluations are still needed to determine the best treatment options. To date, very little empirical research has been conducted to assess the effectiveness of therapeutic modalities for trafficked youth.

There are several psychotherapeutic approaches identified for the treatment of sexual abuse in children and adolescents that may also be appropriate for commercially sexually exploited youth. In fact, many of the treatment recommendations for trafficked youth come from programs used to treat other victimized groups, including victims of sexual abuse, domestic violence, and torture, and from organizations who work with sexually exploited youth. More research is needed to determine the most efficacious mental health treatment. Overall, however, there is general consensus that a multidisciplinary, trauma-informed approach embedded within a system of care model is needed.

General Principles Include Using a Multidisciplinary Approach and Trauma-Informed Care

Given the complex legal, social, and medical/mental health needs of commercially sexually exploited youth, a coordinated multiagency approach is important to fully address the needs of this population. A systematic review of the literature addressing the needs of international survivors of sex traffickers summarized 4 key components of care: starting with a comprehensive needs assessment of survivors, assuring safety and confidentiality, delivering trauma-informed care, and providing comprehensive case coordination.[29] Other experts also highlight the need to effectively educate and train all staff on the complex needs of trafficked youth.[30]

Trauma-informed services have been recognized as a promising approach to providing care in systems such as homeless shelters, the juvenile justice system, and medical settings where sexually exploited youth may present for services. A trauma-informed approach recognizes the symptoms of trauma, understands the impact of past trauma on an individual's life and coping, and incorporates this understanding into practices to empower and avoid retraumatizing the individual.[31] Implementing a trauma-informed model of care can improve identification, diminish harm, and enhance care of youth who have been sexually exploited and victimized.[26,29]

Evidence-based Treatment of Symptoms Associated with Commercial Sexual Exploitation of Children

Although there are not specific evidence-based treatments for youth who have been commercially sexually exploited, mental health treatment of these youth should focus on treating the mental health symptoms with current evidence-based modalities. For youth with PTSD, the most studied treatment is cognitive behavioral therapy (CBT), shown to effectively treat trauma, including exposure to community violence and exposure to trauma among immigrant youth.[32–34] CBT focuses on the interconnectedness of thoughts, behaviors, emotions, and physiologic responses.[35] One promising randomized controlled trial of trauma-focused CBT (TF-CBT), delivered to sexually exploited girls in the Democratic Republic of Congo, demonstrated a reduction in trauma symptoms, decreased anxiety and depression, and improved prosocial behavior. This treatment was culturally adapted, group-based, and delivered by trained facilitators without a mental health background. The authors of this study suggested that part of the positive findings arose from the peer support provided by those with similar experiences.[36] Although this study took place in the Congo with war-affected youth, it has important implications for culturally adapting TF-CBT for populations other than the original intended population, such as for commercially sexually exploited youth in the United States.

There are several other potential evidence-based modalities that could be potentially adapted for trafficked youth. One is multisystemic therapy (MST), a model that takes an ecological approach to treatment and includes the client, the client's family, school, friends, and social services advocates. Originally designed to treat antisocial behavior, MST engages multiple systems to facilitate care of the patient.[35] Dialectical behavioral therapy (DBT), which has been used to treat victims of domestic violence and childhood sexual abuse, may also be beneficial for sexually exploited youth.[37] The cornerstone of DBT involves learning skills of distress tolerance, mindfulness, and emotion regulation, all of which may be especially helpful for youth struggling with self-harming behaviors and maladaptive coping mechanisms.

As there are no current guidelines for the treatment of commercially sexually exploited youth, both pharmacologic and psychotherapeutic treatment of sexually exploited youth should be tailored to the patient and based on the patient's primary and secondary mental health needs, including substance abuse treatment.

Programmatic Interventions

Along with the need for both medical and mental health treatment, many sexually exploited youth are also in need of supportive services and life-skills training. Often youth become involved in commercial sexual exploitation before completing educational training; this can result in a lack of financial, educational, leadership, and self-efficacy skills, and for some, the inability to develop meaningful activities and hobbies. Several programs that provide services to sexually exploited youth have attempted to deliver a more extensive, holistic approach to treatment by teaching these types of skills to commercially sexually exploited youth. In 2007, Clawson and Grace[38] evaluated 4 residential facilities dedicated to serving trafficked youth in the United States, including Girls Educational and Mentoring Services, Transition to Independent Living Program, Standing Against Global Exploitation, Children of the Night, and Angela's House. Although the programs were not formally evaluated with a set of quality metrics, the researchers interviewed key providers delivering services to trafficked youth and identified common elements recommended for residential facilities. These common elements included hiring staffers with specific expertise serving trafficked youth (with some providers advocating prioritizing hiring of survivors), providing intensive case management, life skills, and job training, youth development, family reunification, and education, among others. More formal evaluation of the programs and associated outcomes are needed to determine the best ways to deliver services to these youth and to help guide future development of programs in a trauma-informed, strengths-based framework.

ADDITIONAL RESOURCES FOR PROVIDERS

Commercially sexually exploited youth may have extensive financial, social, legal, immigration, and even basic necessities that often extend beyond a clinician's clinical repertoire. Nevertheless, despite what many trafficked youth have endured, many are resilient and can thrive with appropriate, comprehensive care. Therefore, it is important for psychiatrists and other mental health providers to work in a multidisciplinary, team-based environment in conjunction with service agencies to provide the most thorough care for these youth. In addition, mental health professionals must comply with state child abuse mandatory reporting laws. If a provider does not think that there are adequate resources and support available in their practice or agency, it may be helpful to contact local child protection agencies, or the National Human Trafficking Resource Center, which has a 24-hour hotline available for assistance (**Table 1**). Additional resources, including helpful phone numbers and Web sites, are included in **Table 1**.

Table 1
Trafficking resources

Resources	Web Site	Hotline
National Human Trafficking Resource Center Hotline	http://www.traffickingresourcecenter.org/	1-888-373-7888
National Center for Missing and Exploited Children	http://www.cybertipline.com/	1-800-THE-LOST
Additional information and resources		
Polaris Project	http://www.polarisproject.org/	
Resources for Emergency Healthcare Providers	http://www.humantraffickinged.com/	
Shared Hope International	http://sharedhope.org/	

Finally, there is a role for psychiatrists and other clinicians to advocate for the rights and needs of their commercially sexually exploited patients, which begins with referring to these youth as victims/survivors when communicating with authorities, laypeople, and agencies. Despite Safe Harbor laws and the recognition of trafficked youth as victims under the TVPA, many professionals and members of the general public may still refer to youth as delinquents and may not understand the victim-centered, trauma-informed needs of this population. By raising awareness and educating others, psychiatrists and other mental health providers can contribute greatly to changing policies and treatment practices for this still marginalized group.

SUMMARY

Youth who have been commercially sexually exploited are at high risk for mental health problems, including depression, PTSD, and substance use, given their potential exposure to violence and trauma, as well as difficult and often dangerous living situations. Although youth often do not self-identify as trafficked victims, mental health providers may encounter these youth in various health care settings as well as in juvenile justice and child welfare settings. Child psychiatrists and other mental health providers can serve an important role in identifying, raising awareness, and providing needed mental health services to these youth. Despite the psychosocial adversities and associated mental health and physical health sequelae described in this article, many sexually exploited youth have successfully exited sex trafficking, with some becoming influential advocates who support other sexually exploited survivors. By partnering with advocacy organizations and agencies, and by providing excellent clinical care, child psychiatrists and other mental health providers can help improve the emotional well-being and lives of these youth.

REFERENCES

1. Estes RJ, Weiner NA. The commercial sexual exploitation of children in the US, Canada and Mexico. Philadelphia: Center for the Study of Youth Policy, University of Pennsylvania, School of Social Work; 2002. Available at: http://www.hawaii.edu/search/index.php?cx=008945998903415758105%3A4nrwh9-26ni&cof=FORID%3A11&q=estes+AND+The+commercial+sexual+exploitation+of+children+in+the+US%2C+Canada+and+Mexico&submit.x=7&submit.y=10. Accessed May 5, 2015.

2. West Coast Children's Clinic. Research-to-action: sexually exploited minors needs and strengths. 2012. Available at: http://www.westcoastcc.org/research-to-action-sexually-exploited-minors-needs-and-strengths/. Accessed December 16, 2013.
3. Hossain M, Zimmerman C, Abas M, et al. The relationship of trauma to mental disorders among trafficked and sexually exploited girls and women. Am J Public Health 2010;100(12):2442–9.
4. Zimmerman C, Hossain M, Yun K, et al. Stolen smiles: a summary report on the physical and psychological health consequences of women and adolescents trafficked in Europe. 2006. Available at: http://www.lshtm.ac.uk/php/ghd/docs/stolensmiles.pdf. Accessed November 20, 2013.
5. United Nations Human Rights. Protocol to prevent, suppress and punish trafficking in persons, especially women and children, supplementing the United Nations Convention against transnational organized crime. 2000. Available at: http://www.unodc.org/pdf/crime/a_res_55/res5525e.pdf. Accessed May 30, 2015.
6. United States Government. Trafficking Victims Protection Act (TVPA) of 2000. Vol Pub. L. No. 106–386 Division A, § 103(8)2000.
7. IOM (Institute of Medicine), NRC (National Research Council). Confronting commercial sexual exploitation and sex trafficking of minors in the United States. Washington, DC: The National Academies Press; 2013.
8. Smith LA, Healy-Vardaman S, Snow MA. The national report on domestic minor sex trafficking: America's prostituted children. Shared Hope International; 2009. Available at: http://sharedhope.org/wp-content/uploads/2012/09/SHI_National_Report_on_DMST_2009.pdf. Accessed May 25, 2015.
9. Goodman M, Laurence J. Child trafficking victims and the state courts. In: A guide to human trafficking for state courts. Denver (CO): Human Trafficking and the State Courts Collaborative; 2014. p. 77–88. Available at: http://www.htcourts.org/wp-content/uploads/Full_HTGuide_desktopVer_140902.pdf. Accessed May 8, 2015.
10. Greenbaum VJ. Commercial sexual exploitation and sex trafficking of children in the United States. Curr Probl Pediatr Adolesc Health Care 2014;44(9):245–69.
11. Geist D. Finding safe harbor: protection, prosecution, and state strategies to address prostituted minors. Legis Policy Brief 2012;4(2):67–127.
12. Safe Harbour for Exploited Children Act, N.Y. Soc. Serv. Law §§ 447 A-B.
13. Polaris Project. 2014 state ratings on human trafficking laws. Polaris; 2014. Available at: http://www.polarisproject.org/what-we-do/policy-advocacy/national-policy/state-ratings-on-human-trafficking-laws. Accessed May 22, 2015.
14. McLeroy KR, Bibeau D, Steclker A, et al. An ecological perspective on health promotion programs. Health Educ Q 1988;15:351–77.
15. Reid JA. Entrapment and enmeshment schemes used by sex traffickers. Sex Abuse 2014. [Epub ahead of print].
16. Anderson PM, Coyle KK, Johnson A, et al. An exploratory study of adolescent pimping relationships. J Prim Prev 2014;35(2):113–7.
17. Roe-Sepowitz DE. Juvenile entry into prostitution: the role of emotional abuse. Violence Against Women 2012;18(5):562–79.
18. Curtis R, Terry K, Dank M, et al. Commercial sexual exploitation of children in New York City, volume one: The CSEC population in New York City: size, characteristics, and needs (NIJ Doc. No. 225083). Washington, DC: US Department of Justice; 2008.
19. Stoltz JA, Shannon K, Kerr T, et al. Associations between childhood maltreatment and sex work in a cohort of drug-using youth. Soc Sci Med 2007;65:1214–21.

20. Seng MJ. Child sexual abuse and adolescent prostitution: a comparative analysis. Adolescence 1989;24(95):665.
21. Cole J, Sprang G, Lee R, et al. The trauma of commercial sexual exploitation of youth: a comparison of CSE victims to sexual abuse victims in a clinical sample. J Interpers Violence 2014. [Epub ahead of print].
22. Cochran BN, Stewart AJ, Ginzler JA, et al. Challenges faced by homeless sexual minorities: comparison of gay, lesbian, bisexual, and transgender homeless adolescents with their heterosexual counterparts. Am J Public Health 2002;92(5):773–7.
23. Gwadz MV, Gostnell K, Smolenski C, et al. The initiation of homeless youth into the street economy. J Adolesc 2009;32(2):357–77.
24. Holger-Ambrose B, Langmade C, Edinburgh LD, et al. The illusions and juxtapositions of commercial sexual exploitation among youth: identifying effective street-outreach strategies. J Child Sex Abus 2013;22(3):326–40.
25. Family Violence Prevention Fund. Turning pain into power: trafficking survivors' perspectives on early intervention strategies. Futures Without Violence; 2005. Available at: http://www.futureswithoutviolence.org/turning-pain-into-power-trafficking-survivors-perspectives-on-early-intervention-strategies. Accessed November 21, 2013.
26. Clawson HJ, Salomon A, Grace LG. Treating the hidden wounds: trauma treatment and mental health recovery for victims of human trafficking. Washington, DC: Dept of Health and Human Services; 2007.
27. Greenbaum J, Kellogg N, Isaac R, et al. The commercial sexual exploitation of children: the medical provider's role in identification, assessment, and treatment: APSAC practice guidelines. Chicago: American Professional Society on the Abuse of Children (APSAC); 2013.
28. Muftic LR, Finn MA. Health outcomes among women trafficked for sex in the United States: a closer look. J Interpers Violence 2013;28(9):1859–85.
29. Macy RJ, Johns N. Aftercare services for international sex trafficking survivors: informing U.S. service and program development in an emerging practice area. Trauma Violence Abuse 2011;12(2):87–98.
30. Williamson E, Dutch N, Clawson H. Evidence-based mental health treatment for victims of human trafficking. Washington, DC: US Department of Health and Human Services; 2010.
31. Elliott DE, Bjelajac P, Fallot RD, et al. Trauma-informed or trauma-denied: principles and implementation of trauma-informed services for women. J Community Psychol 2005;33(4):461–77.
32. Cohen JA, Bukstein O, Walter H, et al. Practice parameter for the assessment and treatment of children and adolescents with posttraumatic stress disorder. J Am Acad Child Adolesc Psychiatry 2010;49(4):414–30.
33. Kataoka SH, Stein BD, Jaycox LH, et al. A school-based mental health program for traumatized Latino immigrant children. J Am Acad Child Adolesc Psychiatry 2003;42(3):311–8.
34. Stein BD, Jaycox LH, Kataoka SH, et al. A mental health intervention for schoolchildren exposed to violence: a randomized controlled trial. JAMA 2003;290(5): 603–11.
35. Saunders BE, Berliner L, Hanson RF. Child physical and sexual abuse: guidelines for treatment (revised report: April 26, 2004). Charleston (SC): National Crime Research and Treatment Center; 2004.
36. O'Callaghan P, McMullen J, Shannon C, et al. A randomized controlled trial of trauma-focused cognitive behavioral therapy for sexually exploited, war-affected Congolese girls. J Am Acad Child Adolesc Psychiatry 2013;52(4):359–69.

37. Bohus M, Dyer AS, Priebe K, et al. Dialectical behaviour therapy for post-traumatic stress disorder after childhood sexual abuse in patients with and without borderline personality disorder: a randomised controlled trial. Psychother Psychosom 2013;82(4):221–33.
38. Clawson HJ, Goldblatt LG. Finding a path to recovery: residential facilities for minor victims of domestic sex trafficking. Washington, DC: US Department of Health and Human Services; 2007.
39. Dovydaitis T. Human trafficking: the role of the health care provider. J Midwifery Womens Health 2010;55(5):462–7.

Community-Based Alternatives to Incarceration and Assessment and Community-Based Planning for Probation/Community-Based Alternative

Dalia N. Balsamo, MD*, Yann B. Poncin, MD

KEYWORDS

- Community-based alternatives to incarceration • Adjudicated youth
- Juvenile offenders • Community-based planning
- Evidence-based psychosocial treatments

KEY POINTS

- Incarceration of delinquents has been shown to be costly and detrimental to youth.
- There are several evidenced-based or promising practices that serve youth at risk of incarceration and provide an alternative to incarceration.
- Those with the best evidence for success and those more widely known are reviewed here, and include functional family therapy (FFT), multidimensional treatment foster care (MFTC), multisystemic therapy (MST), and multidimensional family therapy (MDFT).

BACKGROUND

There is growing concern regarding the current treatment of juvenile offenders within the justice system. Although most mental health professionals would agree that it is best to adopt a rehabilitative approach toward delinquent youths, current practices do not always follow this principle. Incarceration has been shown to have a tremendous toll on youth, ranging from their mental health to their educational needs.[1] There are several factors that contribute to the incarceration of youth with mental health

Disclosure Statement: The authors have nothing to disclose.
Child Study Center, Yale School of Medicine, 230 South Frontage Road, New Haven, CT 06519, USA
* Corresponding author.
E-mail address: dalia.balsamo@yale.edu

Child Adolesc Psychiatric Clin N Am 25 (2016) 123–128
http://dx.doi.org/10.1016/j.chc.2015.08.005 **childpsych.theclinics.com**
1056-4993/16/$ – see front matter

problems, including the underdetection of serious mental illness and limitations in treatment availability and quality.[2]

Because of developing concerns regarding the overgrowing use of institutionalized care for children and adolescents, Congress funded the Child and Adolescent Service System Program in 1984. This helped children with mental health needs to access services without necessarily involving the juvenile justice system or child protective services. The Child and Adolescent Service System Program was based on a systems of care approach, which focuses on the child and family's needs, community-based service, and culturally competent care.[3] Although there is an increasing need for mental health treatment for juvenile offenders, community resources and alternatives to incarceration are diminishing, as are financial resources for treatment and rehabilitation programs. There is growing advocacy for juvenile justice reform and mental health research for juvenile offenders.[4] The three most common outcomes following the arrest of a juvenile are (1) official processing through the court system, (2) release with referral for services, or (3) diversion from the system to a variety of community-based services. Although there are evidence-based programs available to juvenile offenders, fewer than 5% are treated with such services on an annual basis.[5]

Evidence-Based Psychosocial Treatments

There are several evidence-based psychosocial treatments that have shown to effectively reduce juvenile criminal behavior in randomized, controlled studies.[6] Three of these evidence-based interventions meet criteria to be designated as model programs in the prevention of delinquency, violence, and drug use by the Blueprints project, developed by the Center for the Study and Prevention of Violence and the University of Colorado Boulder: functional family therapy (FFT), multisystemic therapy (MST), and multidimensional treatment foster care (MTFC).[7] These programs have been implemented outside the United States, such as in Sweden.[8] In addition to these programs, multidimensional family therapy (MDFT) and the MDFT detention to community (DTC) model are discussed in this article as another modality that has demonstrated a significant effect in reducing juvenile criminal behavior. Successfully implementing these community-based treatments is challenging and highly dependent on numerous factors, such as effective training, therapist compatibility, adequate supervision, a solid referral process, available funding, and stakeholder support (**Table 1**).[9]

Table 1
Blueprints model community-based programs for delinquency prevention

Name	Treatment Duration	Treatment Team	Target Population	Blueprints Rating
Functional family therapy	3–4 mo	3–8 Masters-level therapists	Adolescents, all gender and ethnicities	Model
Multidimensional treatment foster care	6–9 mo	10 MTFC parents, family therapist, program supervisor, youth therapist, behavior support specialist, foster parent trainer, and recruiter	Adolescents, all gender and ethnicities	Model
Multisystemic therapy	3–5 mo	3–4 Masters-level therapists, program supervisor (Master's or Doctorate level)	Adolescents, all gender and ethnicities	Model Plus

FUNCTIONAL FAMILY THERAPY

FFT occurs in several treatment phases: engagement, motivation, relational/interpersonal assessment and change planning, behavior change, and generalization/eco-systemic integration.[10] Its ecological approach takes into account the various environmental influences on the youth's behavior, such as family, peer network, school system, and neighborhood. Studies have shown a higher degree of recidivism in adjudicated youth receiving FFT in a community juvenile justice setting 12 months posttreatment compared with probation services. This outcome depended on therapist adherence to the model.[11]

Functional Family Parole: Combining Functional Family Therapy with Probation Supervision

Functional family parole is an adapted version of FFT, which was originally developed in the state of Washington. It integrates the principles of FFT into a probation supervision model. Probation officers are actively involved in delivering the functional family parole model to youth and their families. Studies have shown that youth receiving FFT had fewer out-of-home placements than matched comparisons during the first 2 months after release, although the rates between the two groups were similar by 36 months.[12]

MULTIDIMENSIONAL TREATMENT FOSTER CARE, ALSO KNOWN AS TREATMENT FOSTER CARE OREGON

MTFC was initially developed in Oregon and places at-risk youth in well-trained and supervised foster homes. As in many other in-home models, MTFC is strength-based and builds on positive reinforcement. Focus is on training and supporting the foster parents; providing individual therapy to the youth; and work with other systems, such as school. In general, MTFC placements last between 6 and 9 months. There are four key elements that are addressed in MTFC: (1) providing the youth with positive reinforcement, (2) providing clear limits and structure, (3) providing close supervision, and (4) fostering positive peer relationships for MTFC youth while avoiding harmful ones.[13] The treatment team usually works with 10 cases at a time. They typically include 10 MTFC families, one full-time program supervisor, one part-time family therapist, one part-time youth therapist, and an hourly skills trainer. The youth therapist acts as the youth advocate with no limit setting, whereas the program supervisors function as rule enforcers. Skills trainers are either behavior support specialists, who aid the youth in developing more prosocial behaviors, or foster parent trainers and recruiters. This particular set-up helps to ensure a treatment plan that supports and disciplines youth as needed.[13] Some studies have shown that youth who participated in MTFC reported significantly fewer criminal activities and had significantly lower criminal referrals compared with youth participating in group care.[14] A recent study has shown that MTFC has been effective in reducing delinquency in female juvenile offenders.[15]

MULTISYSTEMIC THERAPY

As its name indicates, MST aims to target risk factors across multiple system levels (family, school, community). It is a home-based program that strives to empower caregivers in obtaining the necessary skillset to effectively parent their children. Treatment lasts from 3 to 5 months, and is quite intensive, 60 or more hours of direct contact with family or other members of the youth's community.[16] Although it does not follow a fixed manualized approach, it is based on a set of treatment principles.

Mutisystemic Therapy Adaptations

MST has been adapted to address other issues and conditions. For example, MST for youth with problem sexual behavior focuses on the ecological factors contributing to juvenile sexual delinquency.[16] Other adaptations include MST for substance abuse, MST for child abuse and neglect, and MST for juvenile drug court, among others.[17] MST for substance abuse combines MST principles with contingency management. Contingency management is an evidence-based treatment model in targeting substance abuse. Studies have shown that it is superior to standard MST for adolescents suffering from substance abuse.[18] A recent study from the United Kingdom demonstrated that the MST model was superior in reducing offending and antisocial behavior when compared with other evidence-based interventions.[19]

MULTIDIMENSIONAL FAMILY THERAPY

Although MDFT is not traditionally listed as a community-based treatment of adjudicated youth, it has been shown to decrease delinquent behavior and affiliation with delinquent peers when compared with control subjects.[20] MDFT attends to four main intervention areas: (1) the adolescent; (2) the parents and/or guardians; (3) the family; and (4) the extrafamilial systems, such as schools. In a DTC study, youth receiving MDFT were detained fewer days than youth receiving regular services.[20] They also received less punitive dispositions.

Multidimensional Family Therapy: Detention to Community

A DTC study tested a two-stage cross-system (substance use and juvenile justice) adaptation to MDFT, which also included a human immunodeficiency virus/sexually transmitted disease prevention intervention. The first stage of MDFT-DTC is in-detention and the second stage is postdetention and community-based. Although the integrative model proved to be successful, no funds were available to sustain it beyond the study.[21]

CASE VIGNETTE: MULTIDIMENSIONAL FAMILY THERAPY

Jake is a 16-year-old boy with trauma in his early life from domestic violence between his mother and birth father. He currently lives with his mother, mother's husband, and their daughter, his half-sister. He has had sporadic contact with his father over the years and his father is currently out of state and uninvolved. Jake was arrested for disorderly conduct and breach of peace on two separate occasions and spent a week in detention. He has used drugs on and off for 2 years, beginning with marijuana and experimenting with alcohol and other street drugs. Jake was referred to MDFT to address his substance use, oppositional behavior, stealing at home, school avoidance/truancy, and intrafamily conflict.

In Stage One of MDFT (Building the Foundation and Multiple Therapeutic Alliances) the clinician explores Jake's motivation for treatment, establishes a collaborative process, and gets to know Jake's life in detail in a strength-based manner. He learns about Jake's interest in music and his daily commitment to writing lyrics and songs. With the parents, the therapist explores their stress and concerns and their past efforts. He looks back to a time where the parents saw a more positive relationship, and he reinforces the notion to the parents that "you are the medicine" for Jake getting better. In the Parent Relationship/Family Interaction Module of Stage One, the therapist assesses family interactions, including how Jake's family talks to one another and the warmth and love in the relationship. Jake's mother and stepfather are at their "wit's end" with Jake, blaming him for the family turmoil. They use harsh, sarcastic language with little praise for expected behavior, saying, "He should do what he needs to do and not expect thanks." Meanwhile the team (clinician and therapist assistant) also collaborate with Jake's school to obtain records, and speak to the probation officer to better understand expectations. A drug screen is administered, which shows positive findings for THC.

In Stage Two and Three (Working the Themes and Requesting Change) the components of the earlier stage are carried over and therapy proceeds. There are several therapeutic goals and strategies, including preparing Jake to talk about important issues with his parents and having him examine his own behaviors in an honest way and the consequences of such behaviors. He recognizes, for example, that he has lost close friends over his legal and drug issues. He is worried about his future because of missed school, but also plays it off as "no big deal." At the same time, the therapist prepares Jake's parents to truly listen to Jake without "flipping out." The therapist also works on the parents' own hopes and expectations for themselves and explores their parenting conflicts. Jake's mother discusses her own trauma and harsh upbringing and the parents discuss their open disagreement about how to deal with Jake's behaviors. In the family work, the conflict with Jake is brought out into the open, so it can be worked on, while the family is also helped to regulate their affect when in session. Jake had been initially unable to remain in the room with his parents to discuss any of his difficulties, but as the family sessions become safer and calmer, he feels more free to voice his concerns. Likewise his mother expresses herself without Jake rolling his eyes or bringing up past injustices. The stepfather learns to support his wife, backing her up, without resorting to denigrating language with Jake.

In Stage Three (Seal the Deal and Exit) the changes and progress that have been made are openly acknowledged, and thoughts and feelings about ending treatment are explored. Jake is still using marijuana but less frequently. He is attending school again on a regular basis, and he has reconnected with an old friend. He has stayed out of further legal difficulties, and the probation officer expects that probation will end after Jake completes community service hours, which he has been doing satisfactorily. Jake's parents observe that they feel more capable about handling what they now see as "typical teenage" behaviors. Jake's mother has decided to pursue her own treatment, having recognized that her own history continues to affect her reactions in the family. These ongoing difficulties are "on the table" and thus easier to tolerate for Jake and his parents, and all agree that they have the ability now to work through any emerging problems.

SUMMARY

There are several program models available to serve youth at risk for incarceration. These models generally have in common the expectation that therapists follow a manualized approach or an approach embedded in firm principles. Therapist supervision and training are closely monitored with many models also including supervision of supervisors, thus ensuring a quality feedback loop at all levels of care-delivery. This ensures model fidelity and that the care delivered remains tethered to the evidence supporting it. Population-specific models such as these, which are closely aligned with care principles, also allow for an expertise to emerge and then inhere within the care team. Evidence-based programs often demand more from funders, and thus their use depends on pubic policy issues, cost-benefit analyses (including present vs delayed costs), and other funding and stakeholder decisions rather than their clinical utility alone.

REFERENCES

1. Lambie I, Randell I. The impact of incarceration on juvenile offenders. Clin Psychol Rev 2013;33:448–59.
2. Erickson CD. Using systems of care to reduce incarceration of youth with serious mental illness. Am J Community Psychol 2012;49:404–16.
3. Poncin Y, Woolston J. Systems of care, wraparound services, and home-based services. In: Dulcan MK, editor. Dulcan's textbook of child and adolescent psychiatry. Arlington (VA): American Psychiatric Publishing, Inc; 2010. p. 925–38.
4. Thomas CR, Penn JV. Juvenile justice mental health services. Child Adolesc Psychiatr Clin N Am 2002;11:731–48.

5. Hengeller SW, Schoenwald SK. Evidence-based interventions for juvenile offenders and juvenile policies that support them. Soc Policy Rep 2011;25(1):3–20.
6. Sukhodolsky DG, Ruchkin V. Evidence-based psychosocial treatments in the juvenile justice system. Child Adolesc Psychiatr Clin N Am 2006;15:501–16.
7. Available at: blueprintsprograms.com. Accessed May 15, 2015.
8. Gustle LH, Hansson K, Sundell K, et al. Blueprints in Sweden. Symptom load in Swedish adolescents in studies of functional family therapy (FFT), multisystemic therapy (MST) and multidimensional treatment Foster care (MTFC). Nord J Psychiatry 2007;61:443–51.
9. Henggeler SW, Sheidow AJ. Empirically supported family-based treatments for conduct disorder and delinquency in adolescents. J Marital Fam Ther 2012;38(1):30–58.
10. Alexander JF, Robbins MS. Functional family therapy: a phase-based and multicomponent approach to change. In: Murrihy RC, Kidman AD, Ollendick TH, editors. Clinical handbook of assessing and treating conduct problems in youth. New York: Springer Science + Business Media, LLC; 2010. p. 245–71.
11. Sexton T, Tuner C. The effectiveness of functional family therapy for youth with behavioral problems in a community practice setting. J Fam Psychol 2010;243(3):339–48.
12. Darnell AJ, Schuler MS. Quasi-experimental study of functional family therapy effectiveness for juvenile justice aftercare in a racially and ethnically diverse community sample. Child Youth Serv Rev 2015;50:75–82.
13. Chamberlain P. The Oregon multidimensional treatment foster care model: features, outcomes, and progress in dissemination. Cogn Behav Pract 2003;10(4):303–12.
14. Chamberlain P, Reid JB. Comparison of two community alternatives to incarceration for chronic juvenile offenders. J Consult Clin Psychol 1998;66(4):624–33.
15. Leve LD, Chamberlain P, Smith DK, et al. Multidimensional treatment foster care as an intervention for juvenile justice girls in out-of-home care. In: Miller S, Leve LD, Kerig P, editors. Delinquent girls: contexts, relationships, and adaptation. New York: Springer Science + Business Media, LLC; 2012. p. 147–60.
16. Schaeffer CM, McCart MR, Hengeller SW, et al. Multisystemic therapy for conduct problems in youth. In: Murrihy RC, Kidman AD, Ollendick TH, editors. Clinical handbook of assessing and treating conduct problems in youth. New York: Springer Science + Business Media, LLC; 2010. p. 273–92.
17. Available at: www.mstservices.com/files/MSTadaptations.pdf. Accessed May 15, 2015.
18. Zajac K, Randall J, Swenson CC. Multisystemic therapy for externalizing youth. Child Adolesc Psychiatr Clin N Am 2015;24(3):601–16.
19. Butler S, Baruch G, Hickey N, et al. A randomized controlled trial of multisystemic therapy and a statutory therapeutic intervention for young offenders. J Am Acad Child Adolesc Psychiatry 2011;50(12):1220–35.
20. Rowe CL. Multidimensional family therapy: addressing co-occurring substance abuse and other problems among adolescents with comprehensive family-based treatment. Child Adolesc Psychiatr Clin N Am 2010;19(3):563–76.
21. Liddle HA, Dakof GA, Henderson C, et al. Implementation outcomes of multidimensional family therapy-detention to community: a reintegration program for drug-using juvenile detainees. Int J Offender Ther Comp Criminol 2011;55(4):587–604.

Index

Note: Page numbers of article titles are in **boldface** type.

Child Adolesc Psychiatric Clin N Am 25 (2016) 129–138
http://dx.doi.org/10.1016/S1056-4993(15)00099-1 childpsych.theclinics.com

D

E

F

I

J

N

O

V

Y

Z

Printed and bound by CPI Group (UK) Ltd, Croydon, CR0 4YY
08/05/2025
01864680-0005